Teaching
Christian Childbirth

Teaching
Christian Childbirth

By Jennifer Vanderlaan

Birthing Naturally ✦ 2010

Teaching Christian Childbirth
© 2010 Jennifer Vanderlaan
www.birthingnaturally.net
All Rights Reserved

Published 2010 by Birthing Naturally, Colonie NY 12205
ISBN 10 0-9765541-4-3
ISBN 13 978-0-9765541-4-1

For Erin,
First to have the vision for this book;
Friend through the easy and difficult;
Thank you for never giving up.

Contents

Part One

Teaching Basics

Chapter One

Ethical Issues in Teaching Christian Childbirth

From a pure ministry standpoint, a Christian Childbirth class is a fantastic way to meet the spiritual needs of the Christian church and reach out to the hurting in our communities. Pregnancy is a time of self-reflection and may be the first time in a person's life when the question "who do I really want to be?" is answered honestly. Because of this, the time of pregnancy and giving birth is one of the most spiritually fertile times in a woman's life.

Not only does the woman become more focused on who God would have her be, but the family unit as a whole undergoes a dynamic change as they prepare for the arrival of a new soul. The couple evaluates their priorities, their schedules, their eating and health habits, their living situation and every other aspect of their lives because the new child will affect their whole lives. During this time of reflection, the couple can be shepherded into a closer relationship with Christ, or they can be pulled away from Christianity and Christ. Christian Childbirth Education is one more way for a couple to strengthen their faith in God.

Christian Childbirth Education is also a useful evangelistic tool for the community as a whole. A couple who may not be ready to step into a church service may be willing to attend a Christian Childbirth class. A single woman who feels judged by others because she is pregnant may avoid church, but be open to a free childbirth class at a pregnancy center. When the local church is meeting the needs of the community, the community members will seek out the local church. Christian Childbirth Education is just one more way the local church can meet the needs of the community.

It is important to remember that even though the class may be offered as part of a ministry, there are generally accepted standards of practice in the medical community which must be adhered to. There are also laws which regulate who can and can not provide certain types of medical information to the general consumer. In addition, the families your classes will be serving have expectations of the type and quality of information you will be providing. All these factors may seem overwhelming as you begin your childbirth education ministry, but by following the guidelines set out in this chapter, you can have confidence that your education program is of the highest quality.

Medical Standards

The first standard to accept is that it is the right and responsibility of the client to make his or her own decisions. Although we sometimes get a picture in our heads of a person going to the doctor and getting instructions for what to do, that is not quite the way our system is designed to work.

A medical caregiver (doctor or midwife) is hired by the client to offer information which is not available to the client alone. This may be medical tests, x-rays, or treatment options the caregiver has been trained in. The client then takes the information and makes a decision as to how she will proceed. At no time does the caregiver have the right or responsibility to tell the client what to do. The caregiver should not attempt to manipulate or coerce the client into making a certain decision.

This standard carries over into your childbirth classes. At no time do you have the right or responsibility to tell the client how to proceed. As an educator, you will help the client explore options and you may suggest sources of information, but you will never make a decision for the clients you serve. You will also never tell them the "right" way to handle a situation. Even though there may be generally accepted standards of the "right" way to manage birth, you must remember that not every situation is the same, and not every family has the same goals for labor.

Because of this, you must be careful how you present comfort measures, interventions and other aspects of labor the client will need to make a decision about. The general rule is to teach facts, risks and benefits that can be proven through research, rather than discussing opinions. It can take a great deal of faith in God to allow the facts to speak for themselves, because some families will look at the facts and choose to respond differently than you would.

Closely related to this is the standard of informed consent. Informed consent means the client has the right to consent or to refuse any treatment after having been informed of:

- Why the treatment is recommended;
- What the treatment is expected to accomplish;
- What are the risks of the treatment;
- What other options may be available;
- What are the benefits and risks of other options.

Without having the answers to all of these questions, the client is not educated enough to make an accurate decision about how she would like to proceed. When questions are left unanswered, the client does not have a full picture of how her decision can or will affect her health.

In some hospitals, the client is required to sign an informed consent document during labor to acknowledge that she has been informed of her options. Unfortunately, labor is not an easy time for a woman to take in new information and many women become highly compliant to any suggestion during labor. Because of this, it is increasingly the responsibility of the childbirth educator to present the available options to the client so she has the time to research her choices before labor begins.

Teaching Implications of Medical Standards

Because it is the responsibility of only the client to decide how she will proceed with her care, the childbirth educator must be careful to ensure class information is presented in a way that allows the client to learn without coercion to adopt the teacher's opinions. Because the teacher is seen as an authority, her opinions will carry some weight with the client, and some clients may simply adopt the teacher's views without examining their own goals, concerns or opinions. Options are to be presented as option only. There is no situation in which you would tell a client how she "should" proceed.

This can be difficult in a childbirth class because many clients will ask you if they "should" or "can" do something. Clients will want your approval for everything from not taking prenatal vitamins to changing care providers. Unfortunately, you can not allow yourself to answer yes or no to these types of questions. You must train yourself to answer the risks and benefits of the procedure and then ask the client how she feels about it. It is appropriate to remind her that it is her decision and that you can help her find information so she is more comfortable making a decision. However, under no circumstances will you make a decision for a client.

It may be helpful to use the client's hesitation to prompt her to do more self-study. When asked if she "should" do something, a childbirth educator can answer, "It sounds like you feel you need more information to make a decision. Can I suggest some resources that may help you feel more prepared?"

Rather than presenting your opinions on the topics at hand, you will encourage your clients to explore research, their feelings and their concerns. Activities which provide interaction time give clients the opportunity to see a wide range of attitudes on the subject instead of just the teacher's attitude. Interactive sharing times can be a great warm-up activity for a class. You may begin a session on first stage labor by asking the class to "Share the advice that friends, relatives and strangers have given them about labor." Your class will immediately be presented with various beliefs about childbirth. You can then ask them to evaluate the truthfulness and usefulness of these beliefs. In this way, clients begin to challenge themselves to form an honest understanding instead of simply applying the teacher's view to their lives.

Another useful tool is worksheets that require self-reflection such as a self-evaluation on options before writing a birth plan. The very writing of a birth plan can make clients feel there is a "right" answer they must find because most clients will present it to the teacher and to the medical care provider. Giving them the opportunity to speak and write about their feelings and goals before they present them in a birth plan can help the client understand that the "right" information on a birth plan is the information they decide to share, not the information they may have found on a sample birth plan.

Preparing a client for informed consent takes more than what can be provided in a lecture. Most adults remember very little of what they hear, and simply hearing a fact does not mean the client can properly apply that fact. To be truly able to provide informed consent, you must give your clients information about the options available through lecture and reading materials. Then you must give them the ability to apply the information they have. This can be done through mock-labor games that allow the client opportunities to make decisions and explore the possible outcomes of those decisions.

It can be tricky to decide what information to include. With such a wide variety of natural and medical options available to birthing families, most childbirth classes are not able to cover every possibility. For this reason, it is best to focus the class efforts on the most common options, and use the time to teach the clients how to find information about the options available to them. Instead of having clients read an article about epidurals as homework, you may ask them to find three articles about the use of medications in labor. By providing them with the skills to find the information they need, you help them prepare for informed consent on every decision they will need to make.

Another aspect to informed consent is helping the clients understand they can make an informed refusal of any procedure. Simply telling the clients that they have this right does not prepare them to refuse procedures during labor; they need to practice discussing their decisions. A simple way to provide this practice is to let your class debate the pros and cons of common interventions. This works especially well if you have the clients research the interventions before class.

Although you may feel limited that you are not able to share what you think is "right" with your clients, ultimately it will make your classes more beneficial to your clients. Instead of them making decisions because "my teacher told me this was best," their work and research will firmly plant their decisions in their heart and head so they will be better prepared to use them in labor.

Legal Standards

Every community has laws about who may or may not provide medical information to consumers. These laws are designed to protect the general public from poorly educated individuals giving bad advice or performing treatments without adequate training. The medical community takes these laws seriously because they are the only assurance the public has of the integrity of our medical system. To legally practice, a caregiver must provide adequate proof of knowledge and skills.

Although it seems to be obvious that pregnancy is a normal and healthy condition for women, by defining the practice of medicine as the diagnosis and treatment of conditions, it is not necessary for a woman to be ill for your suggestions to be considered medical advice. Pregnancy is a healthy condition for the body to be in, but it is still a condition.

In many communities direct-entry midwives (those who are trained in midwifery without training as nurses first) are limited in their ability to serve because of this designation. As a childbirth educator, you will also be limited in your ability to serve. To prevent conflict with the medical community, be sure that you are only offering education and not diagnosing or treating conditions.

At the time of this writing, there is no national standard for certification as a childbirth educator. There are several programs that will certify individuals who complete a training program, however receiving a certification is not a requirement to teach. Many hospital programs require a certification to teach childbirth classes, and a certification program should be considered an investment in a business. Although it is not necessary to become certified to teach, you should be sure to communicate to your clients the type of training you have had. If the class is good, word of mouth will bring clients regardless of a certification.

Teaching Implications of Legal Standards

For the most part, these laws will not affect your childbirth class. However, you do need to be aware that only licensed health care providers are allowed to diagnose medical conditions and recommend treatments. You are an educator; you only give educational information.

This means when a client comes to you and asks what she can do about heartburn in pregnancy you cannot tell her to "just do this." That would be prescribing treatment for a medical condition. It also means when a client asks you why she is getting a certain kind of back pain you cannot tell her "it sounds like you have…"

Instead, when approached with a personal medical question by a client, you can provide educational information. You may let your client know about one or more sources of information that can help her figure out what it could be. You may suggest she ask her caregiver to help her figure out what it is.

This type of advice giving takes practice to master, but is necessary. Guard your mouth so that you do not misuse your position as childbirth educator. Some good phrases to begin your answer with are:

"Some women have tried ____. Other women find ____ helpful. I could help you find more information about these."

"I have a book (or article) that talks about that. Perhaps you could find some answers there."

"That is a common complaint and could be caused by several things. You could explore these possibilities with your caregiver..."

Training yourself to speak wisely to your students will not only help them take responsibility for their own health, but it will also help to keep you humble. When you are the authority in a subject, it is easy to begin to feel prideful about your knowledge. But the position of childbirth educator is not to be taken as one of social standing or intellectual significance. The most important role of the childbirth educator is to be the servant to expectant families. Your job is to serve their needs and to provide them with resources and information.

A quick review of childbirth forums, chat groups and web sites on the internet will allow you to see that in the area of childbirth, a little knowledge puffs up greatly. Most of these professionals have good intentions of helping clients; however, because they have allowed their intellectual authority to make them prideful, they can come across as pushy, know-it-alls or worse. An attitude of pride screams volumes to clients who will for the most part shut themselves off to the materials presented. No one wants to learn from a know-it-all. Even God opposes the proud, but gives grace to the humble *Proverbs 3:34.*

Client Standards

Your clients will have certain expectations of you as the childbirth educator. They expect you will be professional and your material will be trustworthy. You are educating your clients, and they do have the right to expect that you are well informed on the subject you are instructing. Your learning should be on-going, always looking for new research and new ways to handle labor.

You must also remember that you will have access to more information than most of your students. When they enter your classes, they will

probably have some misconceptions about the process of labor and how to handle it. Your clients expect that they will be educated without feeling judged or humiliated for what they did not know. It is important that you find a way to share information that is unbiased and gentle.

Because you are teaching Christian childbirth classes, your clients may also expect a standard of modesty and accountability with the materials you use. Although we must be realistic to the fact that childbirth does require some element of nudity, the Christian childbirth educator should be sensitive to the moral standards her clients have set for themselves. You should also be sensitive to the non-Christian overtones of some childbirth education materials.

Depending on your client base, you may be expected to provide an experience that will prepare for natural birth or one that prepares for the use of pain medications. You may be expected to incorporate the role of the husband or another loved one, or you may be expected to prepare the woman to labor without support. It is important to know what your clients expect from you.

Your clients' perception of your classes will be the driving force behind the success of your childbirth education ministry. If your clients leave your program dissatisfied, feeling ill-prepared or attacked, they will not recommend your program. It will not take long for word to get out that a program is not worth using. If you want your classes to be well attended, it is vital that you keep the highest level of standards for your client interactions.

Teaching Implications of Client Standards

You must strive for the highest level of professionalism. This means you are prompt, polite and business like when dealing with inquires about your classes, your materials are designed with the reader in mind, and you teach your classes with integrity. Teaching a class is a commitment, and your clients will expect your attendance at every class. Missing classes or canceling a session communicates to your clients that the class is not valuable to you.

The materials you use should be accurate, easy to understand and should label the source. This allows the client to assess the trustworthiness of the information presented and return to the source for answers to additional questions. When possible, provide the references to research you are quoting.

Also, be sure you are respecting the copyright of materials you would like to use in your class. It may seem harmless to just copy an article; however the author does have rights to her intellectual property.

It is usually very easy to contact the author and get permission to make copies for educational use.

As an educator, you are presenting yourself as an expert in childbirth. You should be continually increasing your knowledge of the birth process, available options and the birth community in your area. Tell a client when you do not have an answer to a question, but you should be able to answer most of the questions or at least find the answer in a reasonable amount of time. A good habit is to read a different book about birth every month or two. You may also find it beneficial to subscribe to an online birth newsletter or order a subscription to a childbirth journal.

It is normal to give more weight to information that comes from a reliable source, and your students will do that with the information you give them. Be sure the facts you present are facts and come from research you can verify. It can sometimes be difficult to discern the difference between fact and opinion when reading an article or book, so prayerfully review your sources. Give less weight to authors who back up their arguments with "research shows" or other such comments without citing any specific studies.

If you have not yet, familiarize yourself with a scientific study and how to read one. Become comfortable with the format of a study; it is designed in a way that makes it easy for the reader to find the information she is looking for. If you have access to the internet, start searching the Cochrane Review web site at www.cochrane.org for a large collection of highly reliable scientific studies. You may also find the information at Childbirth Connection, www.childbirthconnection.org, helpful.

You could purchase subscriptions to several birth related journals to find studies, but that may not be necessary. Many libraries, especially university libraries, give their patrons access to online journals for research. Finding research can begin with an online database such as Medline, or you may look through the citations listed in articles and books.

The first part of most studies is the abstract, and for some studies this may be the only part you can access without a subscription to the journal in which it is published. The abstract is a type of quick review of what the study looked at and what its conclusions were. It can be difficult to determine the validity of a study if you only have access to the abstract.

When reading a study, pay special attention to a few important points. First, are the conclusions drawn from the results consistent with the results and the study as a whole? Researchers are human too, and they can be swayed by their own biases even when trying to do a completely unbiased study. As you read the results and conclusions, ask yourself if there is something missing, or if other explanations have been ignored.

The second thing to look at is the population used in the study. Sometimes the selecting of a population can skew a study one way or the other. Results from a study of teen mothers may not necessarily be applicable to mothers over forty. Look also at the way participants are put into control and research groups. If this were not done randomly but instead based on decisions made during labor, the grouping may mask other factors that influence the outcome of the study.

Another factor to consider is whether the research demonstrates a causation (the presence of A caused B), or a correlation (A and B seem to happen together). Compare the study to other research available to determine if overall the results seem consistent. If the results are not reproducible in other studies, there are very likely some errors in the research.

Teaching Materials

There are a wide variety of teaching materials available for use in your class. Companies produce and sell charts, movies, demonstration models, handouts and collections of activities. As the childbirth educator, it is your responsibility to choose items that reflect the values and needs of your clients.

Some companies will give you the opportunity to review a movie before you purchase it. This allows you to check for language, unnecessary nudity or other activities that may go against the moral values of your clients. It is important to remember a client who feels she is not being respected is less likely to listen to what you have to say, not only for that day, but for the rest of the class series.

Sometimes this will result in a confrontation with a student who challenges your moral values. If this happens, it is important to remember to stay calm. Understand that whether intentional or not, you did offend a sister, and even if her behavior is not very loving as she confronts you about it, she is confronting you because she has been hurt and wants to prevent others from being hurt. For most people, giving an explanation of why you chose that material—as imperfect as it is—while expressing your sincere regret for having hurt them will smooth the ruffled feathers.

Some people with gentle spirits will completely shut off and be unable to participate if they feel their values have been challenged. If this happens, they will probably not tell you, but you will be able to see them withdraw from the group. It is not necessarily that they are judging you, but rather they are feeling judged and as if they do not "fit in." If this happens you will need to be quick to give the students a chance to give feedback about the material, being sure to ask not only what they liked, but what they did not like about it too. Be sensitive to the most gentle of individuals as you select materials.

Client Base

You will be wise to mold your classes to meet the needs of your client base. The way you design your childbirth ministry will reflect the social, spiritual and educational backgrounds of your clients. Your classes will be more effective if you are able to focus on the needs of the group you serve.

If you have designed your ministry to serve women in a crisis pregnancy center, you may find most of your clients come without partners and will need to be educated in ways to have the best possible labor without labor support. This may change the way you do labor rehearsals, which traditionally give the labor partner experience in comfort measures.

If your class serves low income families, you may find the health care provided to them does not offer as many options as the health care provided to a woman with private insurance. If your class serves families with high levels of education, they may have already done a lot of their own research and not want to sit through classes that give information they have already read about.

Always keep the needs of your clients in mind as you design your childbirth classes. If your ministry is large or serves a large population, you may find it helpful to offer different classes to meet specific needs.

Colossians 3:23-24.

Whatever you do, work at it with all your heart, as working for the Lord, not for men, since you know that you will receive an inheritance from the Lord as a reward. It is the Lord Christ you are serving.

Chapter Two

Facilitating Learning

You may be accustomed to thinking of the childbirth educator as a teacher in a typical classroom setting. In this paradigm, the teacher gives the students knowledge which they are then expected to apply. I would like to challenge your thinking a bit here, and ask you to start a mental picture of the childbirth educator as a learning facilitator; not giving the students knowledge, but helping them to develop understanding.

The process of learning is not simply listening to facts at a class. As learners are exposed to new skills, knowledge and ideas, you will find changes in their behavior, attitude and capability. These changes comprise the bulk of learning. As the childbirth educator, you will be providing educational experiences that allow your students to have these types of growth.

Another thing to keep in mind is that as a Christian childbirth educator, you will have the goal of providing the families in your class with an opportunity to meet and fall in love with Jesus. This may or may not affect the way you present material, depending on the make-up of your student body.

Education Basics

There are a few points that may seem almost common sense but should be mentioned at the start because they are also easily overlooked.

First, it is important that you begin at the learner's level. A class of first time mothers who have never been to a labor will need you to teach more basic information than a class of mothers who have been through labor, even if they did not have the experience they had hoped for. Although it is a good idea to review basic information for a review class, the way you present the information will be different.

Secondly, in order for the information to be properly processed, it should be presented in a similar way to how it will be used. For example, if you are teaching massage techniques for comfort in labor, be sure that you have designed a teaching activity that allows the students to actually massage and be massaged.

Another point to remember is that learning takes place with all the senses, not just by hearing or reading. While most adults will only remember 10% of what they read, they will remember 50% of what they hear and see, and 80% of what they hear, see and do. Be sure your activities provide your students with the opportunity to use the skills you are teaching them.

Finally, you must constantly be assessing your students' level of learning. Because the themes in childbirth education build on each other, your students will be left far behind if you move from a topic before they understand the concepts you are trying to teach. After teaching a new skill or giving the students a new knowledge base, present an activity in which they must use the new information in combination with what they have already learned. This allows you an opportunity to determine if they did understand the new material enough to use the information.

Teaching Implications of Education Basics

Functionally, you should strive for a class structure that is dynamic. The activities you choose may change with different class series because each series will be filled with different learners. You may spend more time on one area if a class is having a difficult time with a topic, or you may provide only a short review of a topic if the class already has experience and knowledge of the issue.

Your class structure should also include large amounts of hands-on and student interaction time. Although a lecture is a good way to get a large volume of information into a learner's ears, it does not mean the learner has understood the material enough to make it usable. Additionally, the retention rate for only hearing material is 20%. This means 80% of what you say will not be remembered by the time they attend the next class.

You will need to build assessment activities into your class time. This can be done through rehearsals, practicing skills or a game. Not only will you see if the concepts have been understood, but the class will have more time to practice using the new skills they are learning.

Adult Learning

A good teacher knows her students and understands what they need to learn. You would not get up in front of a class of French-only speaking students and teach a lesson in English because what you would be presenting would be meaningless to them. In the same way, beginning a first-time parent childbirth class with information about medical interventions would be meaningless until they understood the normal labor process. You must adapt your teaching to the student rather than expect the student to adapt to you. For most childbirth classes, the learner will be an adult.

The first thing to know about adult learners is they want to discover something on their own rather than be "taught." This is especially true in some sensitive areas such as nutrition and exercise because being told how to eat can feel like you are being judged. Instead, as the facilitator of learning you must find ways to help your students find the answers they are looking for. Your goal should never be to get your students to have any particular style of birth. Instead it should be to provide your students with the tools to make informed choices about how to handle labor

and birth. Teaching in this way can be more difficult for an educator because it requires the giving up of control. But if you trust the learning process, your students will learn.

Similarly, adult learners like to know they are a part of the decision making process for learning. Expectant parents attend a childbirth class already having beliefs about childbirth and ideas about what they should learn. As a class facilitator, you will quickly realize what they expect to learn is almost always already a part of the syllabus. However, giving them the opportunity to share what they expect to learn with you can help them feel the class has been tailored to their specific needs.

Adult learners will come to your class having a great deal of life experience with which to help them understand the concepts you are presenting. Design activities that engage the students in discovering concepts through experience instead of telling them about concepts. They have already dealt with physically painful or demanding situations and, when asked, can already give you a list of comfort measures to use. They have already made a plan for something, and so should be able to tell you the steps that need to be taken to write a useful birth plan. By drawing on their experiences, you will not only help your students process and retain more information, but you will also build their confidence in their skills and knowledge.

Another key to understanding the adult learner is in general, adults study material because they want to solve a problem, not because they are interested in a subject. In childbirth education, clients will attend your classes not because they want to learn about the birth process, but because they want to know what to do about birth. By planning your classes in a way that gives students specific strategies to improve their birth experience in each class, you encourage them to continue learning through your class.

Finally, for an adult to attend a class, it must have a value specific to her needs. Adults will quickly tire and drop out of a class they feel does not teach them what they need to know. To keep your clients seeing the value of the classes, every class should give them skills for giving birth. This is particularly important for the first class of your series, which clients will use as a test.

Learning Styles

There are many ways individuals learn, and a good childbirth class will provide the students with opportunities to experience learning in all of them. This is in part because each person has a different style of learning with which they are able to learn most efficiently. It is also because what you are teaching involves both information and skills.

The wide varieties of expertise your students develop are necessary for them to plan and achieve the birth they desire. You are not only passing on knowledge, but you are helping your students to develop understanding of the subjects covered, incorporate new skills into the way they handle pain, evaluate their priorities and beliefs, and change their attitudes.

For example, to choose an appropriate comfort measure during labor your class members will need to be able to:

• Recall the normal process of labor
• Determine an appropriate comfort measure
• Physically perform the comfort measure
• Evaluate if the comfort measure is effective

These areas of expertise are all learned in different ways and therefore should be presented in different ways when covered in class. Part of the difference is that the human brain stores information based on the way it was received. Most of us learned the order of the alphabet through a song, which stimulates the right brain (non-dominant part of the brain) and the information is then stored in that area. We learn numerical order as a cognitive, detail item and so it is stored in the left brain (dominant part of the brain).

When you need to recall the information, you must stimulate the part of the brain it is stored in. This is why we can easily and quickly answer a question about what number is before 54, but usually sing to ourselves to figure out what letter comes before L. You need to be aware that the way in which you teach information will affect how the information is stored and how easily your students will recall that information when it is necessary.

In addition to the differences in types of learning, each student in your class will have a way in which she most easily approaches new learning and acquires new information. Individual differences such as whether she learns by trying something or by thinking about something, whether she learns step by step or the big picture easier, whether she needs pictures to see or words to hear, and whether she understands specific facts or by general concepts affect the way students will respond to learning activities. To help your students learn, you must ensure your class offers information in a variety of ways.

In an effort to meet the needs of all your learners, try to ensure that each skill you expect your students to develop is explored in a variety of activities. Give your students opportunities to try out the information and form their own conclusions. This can be completed in the following ways:

1. Give the students a chance to do whatever it is you are trying to help them learn. If you are studying nutrition, let them plan meals or evaluate the nutritive value of meals. If you are studying interventions, allow them opportunities to recommend when the intervention should be used.

2. After trying the new skill, give the students a chance to reflect on the activity, sharing what they learned from the experience. This can be covered through a brief class or small group discussion time after the activity.

3. Ask the students to apply what they have just learned to situations they are likely to face. For example, after trying a few positions for labor and giving the students time to discuss what they liked and did not like about each one, present a labor story and have the students decide what position may be helpful as the labor progresses.

4. Give the students the opportunity to experiment with the new skill after having gained more information. For example, when studying the stages of labor, allow your students to review labor stories and determine when a woman from a story is experiencing the various stages of labor.

In addition to in-class activities, you may want to use homework as a way for students to further experiment with new information. Reading assignments can help them explore new ideas while writing assignments can help them explore their priorities and beliefs about birth. The basic idea is to allow the students access to information from a variety of sources in a variety of ways to ensure each student learns.

Because the goal of the teacher is for the student to use the information shared, the class should be set up in a way that permits the students to be exposed to new ideas, and gain mastery of the new skills presented. Students should be given time to manipulate and practice using the new class materials.

Chapter Three

Teaching Christianity

Mastering a Skill

In Christian childbirth education, you are teaching two skills. One skill is the ability to accurately apply scripture to daily life. The other skill is to give birth. To accomplish this you will need to have a basic understanding of the process of acquiring a skill.

As an example, consider the skill of reading. To truly master reading takes years of experience and many steps. You may begin with an understanding of letters and sounds then move into blending sounds and word identification. Once these basics have been learned, the reader begins to increase eye stamina and reading comprehension. Life experiences help to deepen the understanding of the material. Once mastered, the reader picks up on subtle techniques such as foreshadowing and irony to fully comprehend the authors meaning.

This is the normal process of growth and maturation of a skill. Learning to read is a long process that follows the maturation of each individual. You cannot rush the skills, and you cannot teach the reader to incorporate a technique she is not yet ready for. Yet somehow, by continually practicing the skill of reading, readers learn to assign meaning to a text by the tone as well as the word order.

Experience is not simply the passing of time. As an individual gains experience using a skill, she refines the basic ideas. She makes decisions and learns from her mistakes and her successes. She encounters a wide variety of situations, and begins to understand what is uniquely important to each.

Early in the process of learning a skill, a person may have difficulty. They will rigidly follow "rules" and need to focus attention to make decisions. When the skill is mastered, the "rules" may seem to have been discarded because the decision making process has become a way of looking at the world. This process of improvement at a skill has been explained in the Dryfus Model.

A novice is someone new to the skill. With no practical experience in the skill, the novice must use context-free rules to guide their judgment and performance. The novice is limited and inflexible. There are no grey areas, everything is black and white; right or wrong. The biggest problem facing a novice is that the list of rules does not give information about priorities or the relevance of the rules in specific situations.

An advance beginner is still new to the skill, but has some experience. This experience allows the advanced beginner to identify global characteristics to a situation based on prior experience. The advanced beginner begins to make decisions not just based on the rules, but on prior experience with similar situations.

When a person becomes competent in a skill they have enough experience to be guided by the understanding of a long-range plan or goal. This long-range plan helps her to dictate which rules and aspects of the situation are the highest priority. At this point, she has the feeling of mastery, but may still lack flexibility. She may also take longer to come to conclusions than the more advanced individuals.

The woman who has become proficient has learned to see the situation as a whole rather than a collection of smaller, unrelated parts. As she works toward the long-range goal, the ability to see the whole situation gives her perspective and allows her to quickly assess the priorities. Her personal experiences have given her the ability to predict outcomes. She has a deep understanding of the material.

When someone has mastered a skill, she no longer relies on the rules or principles to connect her understanding of the situation to appropriate actions. She has extensive experience, and may seem to have an intuitive grasp of a situation. She quickly finds the priority actions, but she may not be able to explain why or how. An expert has so mastered the process of decision making, she cannot tell you everything that went into her decision. However, she will still revert to using the basic rules and analytic tools when faced with new situations.

Teaching a Skill

You are somewhere on this continuum for applying scripture to your life, for childbirth, for teaching, for any skill you have tried to learn. Every family you teach will be somewhere on this continuum in terms of their mastery of childbirth skills and their mastery of applying scripture to their lives. Your classes are bound to be populated by individuals at different levels. So, how do you help the novice, the competent and the expert at the same time? The answer lies in using a variety of activities.

Both the novice and the advanced beginner need support and will rely heavily on the "rules" to guide their decisions. You will want to be sure to explain concepts clearly to help beginners understand what the "rule" may be. Move onto a decision making game or a simulation to give practice to those at the competent level. This will also give the beginners a chance to see what the rule looks like in practice.

Those who are proficient will benefit from case studies, which give them an opportunity to see the situation as a whole. Context-free examples may frustrate the proficient who will begin to ask, "What about when...?" Try not to see this as an unproductive behavior, but as the proficient person trying to understand how it all fits together. Experts will still need practice applying their skill to the new situation,

so case studies and decision making games will help them as well

As you work through the material, expect your class members may gain different understandings from the material. Every individual is growing in different areas at different rates, they will not all become expert by attending your class. However, you can expect each individual will have some maturation because of your class. Encourage self-reflection activities to help them see how much growth they have experienced.

In addition to different levels of experience and mastery, each Christian has a unique set of gifts or talents. Spiritual gifting will influence the focus of each class member. This is because an individual's spiritual gift tends to define their first response to a situation. Someone gifted as a servant may first react by meeting physical needs, while someone gifted with a mercy initially focus on the emotional needs. Acknowledging the differences in focus based on our gifts can help to prevent conflict regarding the "right" way to handle a situation.

Mastering the Scriptures

One challenge for the Christian childbirth educator is the interpretation of the Bible. In your class you may have families who have read the Bible daily for twenty years or more sitting next to families who have never picked up a Bible. Even among families with good working knowledge of the Bible you may find differences born of generally accepted societal attitudes and beliefs. How do you know what the Bible says about birth, and what is important to teach?

Before you begin teaching, read through the entire teaching guide and workbook. Take the time to read every scriptural reference. Do not just read the verse, but read the whole passage so you can understand what is being discussed. The concepts taught in the workbook come from the Christian Childbirth Handbook, and it is highly recommended that you read it to help you understand how the material goes together. This will give you a good foundation to understand the material presented in this curriculum.

There are organizations that will train you to teach Christian childbirth. You may find this training helpful in creating an overall philosophy of childbirth from the Christian perspective. Training will also expose you to additional concepts not included in this guide. You have access to a digital copy of the workbook and a variety of handouts at the teaching web site. Take the time to work through the study guides, testing your ability to explain the concepts. Make notes in the sides of this guide as to how you want to incorporate different ideas. Become involved **13** in groups to discuss your thoughts and form your own philosophy of birth.

You have been beautifully and amazingly created by God with your unique combination of gifts and talents. This is blended with your personal experiences and growth in Christ. No two teachers will approach the material the same. No two teachers will highlight the same concepts and principles. What is most amazing, is that this is how God has orchestrated it. God created you to be the person he needed you to be to fulfill his purposes. He will direct the people to your classes who need to hear the message you have to share.

Teaching the Scriptures

You can spend years studying the Bible, and still open it up to learn something new. It is an amazing text; inspired of God; able to speak to you personally regarding your life. Living and active, the Bible is as relevant when you have been a Christian for fifty years as it is when you first become a Christian. The Bible is able to teach and correct, not merely instill knowledge, but build wisdom and inspire action.

The Bible combines history with theory; prophecy with poetry; war with peace. The Bible allows us to see God; to begin to grasp his purposes and to consider his ways. The examples of imperfect people being used in miraculous ways is inspiring; the promises of God are encouraging; the commands of God challenge and motivate us. Jesus taught by quoting scripture. Matthew proved the divinity of Christ by citing scripture. The Pharisees became white washed tombs because of their devotion to scripture.

White washed tombs, what?

It is hard to believe that something as honoring as mastering the scriptures can become a stumbling block. But the truth is, anything done in vain or selfish ambition will separate you from God; even mastering the Bible. The Pharisees did not realize their problem, instead they taught others to follow their ways believing they were honoring God.

To teach Christian childbirth, you must be familiar with the Bible. You need to have a working knowledge of the basic principles of Christianity and you should be aware of passages that relate to fertility and parenting. But be aware of the inherent dangers teaching the scriptures brings with it. James 1:3 warns us of the danger of becoming a teacher—teachers will be judged more strictly.

Teachers spread what they learn. Not simply spreading knowledge, teachers act as mentors to those they teach. The way you make decisions, the way you choose to live your life, the priorities you set, your attitude are all passed on to those you teach.

As such, teachers have the ability to influence the spiritual lives of many more people than they ever come into contact with. This means any sin in your life is multiplied when you are a teacher.

Some Christians struggle with laziness, always doing the least work possible to complete the task. Some Christians struggle with pride, convinced they are always correct. Some Christians struggle with holding others accountable, fearful of making others unhappy or uncomfortable. Some Christians struggle with mercy, unable to see value in expressing ideas in gentler ways. In each of the scenarios, the teacher is at risk of the students accepting her weaknesses as the ideal Christian life.

The difficult reality of teaching Christianity is that who you are is as much a part of the teaching as what you say. There is no secret formula or teaching trick you can use to make this go away. This makes your personal growth one of your highest priorities for being a teacher. You should be in the scriptures regularly, testing yourself against the truth of God. You should have prayer and accountability partners whom you have given permission to speak the truth, even when that truth is uncomfortable to hear. You should have someone you can safely go to with questions and difficult concepts. If at any point you are not where you believe God created you to be, you need to do the work to move yourself back in line with God.

If you can accept the responsibility of a teacher, God can and will perform miracles through your work. If you feel called to teach, but do not yet feel ready, wait. Find the people who will serve as your accountability and prayer partners. Take the time to establish a mentor relationship with the person God reveals to you. Pray and seek God's wisdom. When you are ready and God says begin, go.

When you teach, let the Bible speak for itself. You will notice only the scripture reference is listed in the student workbook. This is to make the students read from the Bible. This way new Christians are able to learn to use the Bible. It allows the Holy Spirit to use the scripture to teach and convict, to grow and mature the members of your class. It helps prevent the "me against you" that can happen when people approach a challenge with different agendas, and helps establish a relationship in which the group works together to figure something out. Most importantly, the spiritual principles are able to be understood as based on God's word rather than simply something the teacher said.

Be ready to give answers when necessary, but be sensitive to the work of the Holy Spirit. It takes patience and discipline to learn to trust God with your class, to give them the freedom to explore ideas and go through the valley before they arrive on the mountain. Sometimes the best answer is another question. Sometimes there are no words you can say. Your job is to provide the opportunity for growth. It is God's job to make the growth happen.

Principles for Childbirth

Christians rarely make decisions based on individual Bible verses. Instead, decisions are made based on Biblical principles; ideas that are supported and developed through the entire Bible. In some cases it is easy to make a decision because the issue is specifically addressed in scripture or one option is supported by all Biblical principles. Other times decisions are more difficult, and individuals must weigh the value of each principle.

The workbook and teacher guide have been written from the perspective of selected Biblical principles. These principles are stewardship, love, faith, freedom, wisdom, peace and children as blessings. You will find a list of verses relating to the main principle explored in each unit on its first page in the workbook. Further discussion on each principle is included in the Christian Childbirth Handbook. It is important that you have a firm understanding of these principles before you begin teaching them. However, this in no way negates the fact that there are other Biblical principles you or families may use to help make decisions. Remember, each individual Christian is a unique combination of experiences, talents and gifts.

The overall theme of the teaching materials in the workbook and handbook are that Christian childbirth is not about what you do, but who you serve. Families seeking God's wisdom and following God's plan may be sent on different paths; one may give birth at home and another may give birth by cesarean. Likewise, two women can have similar birth stories, yet one may have grown closer to God through the experience while the other may have lost her faith.

This may be a difficult concept for some families you teach. Christian childbirth may be likened to Lamaze® or Bradley®, with the expectation you will teach them the proper moves and techniques to give birth in the correct Christian way. Some families may have false understanding of Christian childbirth meaning the birth must be natural, or at home, or unassisted or pain-free to be considered a successful Christian birth. Some families may have been taught that if they have enough faith, everything is guaranteed to go well.

You are unlikely to resolve all the differences of opinion about Christian childbirth that may exist among your class members in just a few short weeks. Remember, entire denominations have been split over disagreement on the importance of various Biblical principles and the interpretation of the Bible. To help you facilitate classes that offer the most opportunity for exploring how the Bible applies to life you will need to make teaching decisions in line with Biblical principles, for example not judging, serving others and accountability.

Jesus is clear in his explanation that no human is in any position to pass judgment on another human being. Humans have a tendency to judge people based on what they can see, however God judges people based on the heart. It is only to his master a servant fails or succeeds. While this does not mean you encourage others to believe lies or misinformation, it does mean you treat them with the dignity and respect a child of God deserves even if you believe they are wrong.

In deciding to teach, you have placed yourself in a position of service to the families of your community. Your job is not to convert families to your way of thinking, but to meet their needs for information, support and encouragement as they grow closer to God through this pregnancy.

Accountability means you ask your students the difficult questions they need to be asked to ensure they are doing the work to grow closer to God. This can be done without pointing out families if you ask your questions well. Instead of asking if families did the reading, ask what they liked or did not like about what they read. Instead of asking if they ate well, ask them what they learned about themselves as they tried to eat better this week. The idea is to ask constructive questions that will help families meet their goals the next week rather than just checking off a to do list.

Chapter Four

The Class as a Group

Unless you are teaching private classes, your childbirth class is a group and will move through the normal stages of a work group. As the class facilitator, you can help your students move through this process easily to allow them the best chance of learning the material presented.

Benefits of Groups

Teaching your class to a group instead of a single couple has several advantages. Foremost is the opportunity the group setting gives your students to interact with other expectant parents, sharing their experiences and building a community. Working in a group allows you the freedom to integrate several active learning strategies, allowing the students to learn from each other.

Students in a group class also benefit from hearing the thoughts and opinions of other class members. This exposure to a variety of philosophies of birth helps to make it acceptable to the expectant parent to define their own philosophy of birthing. The students also find support for the decisions they make with the other members of the class.

Every class you teach will be different. This is because each group of students brings a unique set of skills and experiences to the class. As the teacher, it will be your job to encourage the sharing of these skills and experiences with the class to promote learning in the whole group.

Group Development

Each of us has "groups" in our mind we already belong to. On the first night of class, your students will make mental notes of who is in the same group as them. We have all done this, figuring out where we fit in the group based on who came late, who speaks up and the comments they make. Your students will want to know they are special in your class, and they have something to contribute. It is human nature is to find those differences. It is the role of the group facilitator to help the class members find the ways in which they are similar.

Warm Up Phase

As a group is forming, members pay attention to the group as a whole and determine where they fit. The members look for acceptance by the group and need to know it is a safe place. Their behavior will be predictable, trying to avoid conflicts. Serious topics and feelings are avoided at this time. Class discussion will center around the task at hand.

To move to the next stage, the members of the group must risk sharing thoughts, feeling and ideas about less safe topics. You will set the tone, so greet your students at the door with a friendly smile and ask questions to show you are interested. When your students speak to you, use active listening and be sure to thank them for their contributions to the class.

You will also try to help your students recognize the sameness of their conditions through warm-up discussions and activities. Let them see they are struggling with similar fears, concerns and problems. Allow them opportunities to discover they are all celebrating the same hopes, dreams and wishes. As you introduce new topics, reinforce the universal nature of each subject to help the students form camaraderie. Allow your students adequate time to share in the first few weeks to solidify the feeling of sameness

Work Phase

When the group members feel comfortable with each other, they are able to work together to solve problems and recognize the contributions of all group members. At this stage, members are willing to change their ideas and opinions based on the facts presented by other group members, and will seek information and opinions from each other. At the strongest level, groups in the work phase can easily move from working independently to working in subgroups or within the large group. The group works together to solve problems and there is support for experimenting in solving problems. Creativity is high.

If people feel judged or rejected, they will not contribute to your class discussion. If a student is not comfortable enough to share a problem with the group, you can not give guidance and support. Create an atmosphere of openness—be willing to listen to the thoughts and ideas of class members. Do not always jump to correct misunderstandings, especially if the assumption is about a topic that has not yet been discussed. Encourage other students to share their thoughts and let them know the topic will be discussed during a later class. You may even suggest they begin studying the topic before that class.

Keep a supportive environment for problems and decisions. Lead students to possible solutions without providing the solutions. For example, if a student is having a problem with her care provider, avoid saying "You need to switch doctors." Instead, give the students the tools needed to discover this on their own by asking questions. "Why does your doctor feel that way?" "Is this the only issue you disagree on?" "What have other doctors or midwives told you when you asked for a second opinion?" "Have you taken a copy of that book for your doctor to look at?" "Do you feel comfortable remaining in this doctor's practice?"

You set the tone. If you are closed off, unwilling to listen or share, your students will mirror that. Model active listening for your students. Focus on the individual speaking with your eyes and your mind. Non-verbally acknowledge points in the message,

but stay silent until she is finished. Use your body language to encourage the speaker to continue with her message. Briefly summarize the point; then ask the relevant question or state your idea. Give the speaker time to rest and regroup if necessary before responding to your remarks. Express your appreciation for sharing to help build trust.

At times you may see more garbage than treasure. Some students may only want to complain about everything going on in their lives. You will need to use your strengths (humor, positive attitude, artwork, story-telling), to get the student beyond looking at other peoples problems so they can focus on what needs to be changed in their own life. It will take time for your class to grow to the point that they can work together and learn from each other. Try to plan for a lot of group interaction in the first class or two.

Integration Phase

At the end of the class series, your group members will need to be moved from "student" to "graduate." Ideally, your class will have prepared them to make and act on decisions by giving them the skills they need. Having a planned ending time at the last class for you to recognize students' achievement and to give them an opportunity to say personal good byes can help your group members make the leap from learning the concepts to integrating them into their lives.

You may find it helpful to move your class through the group process at each class. Begin the session with a warm up activity that relates to the topic of the class and requires group input and interaction. Move into the working stage, where your students will actively learn new material. End the session with an integration phase where you review the major points and allow the class to plan how this will be significant in their daily lives.

Unproductive Behaviors

One of the drawbacks of a group is that disruptive and unproductive behaviors affect the entire class. Recognize disruptive or unproductive behaviors and gently correct them before they damage the community.

Poor listeners interrupt or talk while others are presenting information and ideas. A poor listener will cause students or the teacher to feel rejected.

Cynics disagree with everything and everybody no matter what they say. Cynics send a message that opinions and thoughts are unwelcome.

Monopolizers never let anyone else share. They dominate and manipulate the group and sometimes the teacher. Not only do they waste class time, they

17

also prevent the interaction necessary for students to make changes in their attitudes and beliefs.

Show-offs waste group time by telling stories and going off on tangents. They waste valuable class time and energy and prevent the class from moving on to more meaningful topics.

Withdrawers do not participate in activities, and place themselves outside the group. During discussions they may only talk privately. This robs the group of the member's input and prevents the student from learning necessary skills.

Handling Unproductive Behaviors

You can positively handle unproductive behaviors if you remain calm and patient. Do not be defensive; remember the problem is bigger than you. For example, if a person is particularly aggressive, it could be due to a situation at work, not what you are doing. Try to find out more about the problem. It could be there is an additional issue that should be included in the curriculum.

Comment on the behavior without pointing a finger at any one person, and comment at a time other than when the problem is occurring (e.g. at the beginning or end of a session). This will draw the behavior to the members attention and may prevent it from continuing.

Use body language to discourage behaviors, for example, do not make eye contact with a monopolizer. Do not be afraid to turn your back on a student and resume the lesson when she pauses. If a monopolizer continues to talk on and on, gently interrupt and say you appreciate the contribution, and you would like to hear from someone else in the group.

Put withdrawers in small groups where they will feel more comfortable. Identify and make eye contact with the student you would like to answer before you ask questions.

If two participants are constantly talking, stand between them. Give excessive talkers a job to do, such as looking up information, writing notes or drawing an image you need.

Encourage the discussion of cynicism. Getting to the source of participants' lack of confidence in the class's (or their own) ability to make changes can lead to a better understanding of the problems they face

If the problem behavior continues despite all you have tried to discourage it, speak to the person privately. Let the person know how you feel. Tell them how their behavior is affecting you.

Trust the group process. Often, other participants will handle the difficult person themselves.

Chapter Five

Teaching Methods

Choosing a format for presenting new information requires you to understand what the learner is expected to do with the information. Choose the teaching method that gives the learner the best opportunity to master the knowledge or skill.

Lecture

A lecture is an effective way to transfer a large volume of knowledge in a small amount of time. It allows the opportunity to organize material in a way to meet the student's needs. It also gives you the ability to present a complete concept at one time, helping your students see the big picture either before or after other information is given.

However, most individuals are unable to listen effectively to a lecture for a sustained period of time. At least 10 percent of the audience will display signs of inattention after only 15 minutes of lecture. Even if the listeners pay attention, recall after a lecture is very low.

Another problem is lectures are often ineffective at changing attitudes or promoting thought, two necessary components of learning. Although attending a lecture may give you facts and principles, discussion of the material is shown to give the same amount of knowledge while also improving the ability to solve problems and increase student approval of the class.

Students learn best when they are actively involved in the learning process. To make the most of lecture time, incorporate active learning activities such as a short test or quiz after the material is presented; pausing for a few minutes to allow discussion among students; and demonstrating the concepts you are trying to convey. Lectures may also be improved by providing a meaningful way for the students to write or record what is being covered and pausing to give them the opportunity to organize their thoughts in writing.

Examples of lecture topics are the normal labor process, how breast feeding works or how to write a birth plan.

Cooperative Learning

Cooperative learning strategies give the students the freedom to explore new ideas and concepts while still under the guidance of the teacher. Here are some basic formats you can use instead of lecture.

Brainstorming sessions allow the group to share ideas about a topic or answers to a question without worrying about getting the right answer. It is effective at getting class members to discuss attitudes, interests and beliefs about childbirth.

To start a brainstorming session about ways to exercise, you might say, "Tell me all the things a pregnant woman could do to get exercise." Be sure to keep a list of the answers in a place the entire class can see it.

A Buzz Session is when a small group of students is given a limited amount of time to complete a task. It is effective for having the class demonstrate knowledge and understanding of a topic, and can also be used to discuss attitudes, interests and beliefs about childbirth.

To begin a buzz session about nutrition you might say, "Take five to ten minutes with your small group to plan one day of meals following the guidelines for good nutrition."

Guided Discovery happens as the students explore new skills. Students are given a brief explanation and demonstration of the skill. Students then try it themselves. After trying the skill, students will ask questions, answer questions and make observations. This allows you to build on the topic at the students' own pace.

A guided discovery activity for pregnancy exercise may include statements like, "See my feet on the ground and my body leaned forward? This is the squat position. Try it out and tell me how you think this might help you for labor."

Peer Teaching can occur through class presentation of projects or assignments. Students can complete a homework or research assignment and report back to the class. Students can also share what they have learned through small group work with the class as a whole.

To begin peer teaching about childbirth fears you might say, "Last week your homework was to find a movie in which someone gave birth. Did anyone find a movie birth they really liked?"

Debates give the class an opportunity to enhance their skills and understanding while reducing the instructor's biases and forcing the students to deal with their own biases. They can also prompt the students to research topics and improve communication skills. A debate does not need to be a formal presentation to be effective.

To begin a debate about comfort measures you might say, "We're going to have a fun-spirited debate to see just how much we know about these comfort measures. I'm going to give you a labor discomfort. This half of the room will try to convince me to manage it with mental relaxation techniques. This half of the room will try to convince me to use physical relaxation techniques."

Discussion about the class material gives the students the opportunity to share ideas and questions about a topic. The students are able to receive immediate feedback and work together to solve problems with concepts covered in class while they improve their communication skills. There is a sample discussion lesson script on the web site.

Comprehension Activities

Presenting information in a variety of ways can help your students grasp concepts and develop a more thorough knowledge of the topics covered. The following activities can be used to expand your students' understanding.

Webbing is a brainstorming activity in which the class is given a topic and asked to share what they know about it. As the student comes up with ideas, they are added to the web by connecting them to related ideas. This activity can be done by students while watching a movie or as a method of note taking during a lecture.

To begin a webbing exercise, you would hand out paper or the webbing form (available on the web site), and might say. In the center of your web write the words 'healthy pregnancy.' Now fill in your web with all the things you can think of that will help you have a healthy pregnancy. Don't forget to connect the things that are related like avoiding fast food and eating properly."

With **Free Association**, you allow the students to say or write whatever comes to their minds about a topic. It is a great personal exploration, and when used in your class, you can have the students create groups or "clusters" of words that were popular about the topic. You can use free association to help talk about attitudes, values and beliefs about birth or to explore the amount of knowledge the students have on a topic.

To begin a free association activity about nutrition you might say, "What can you tell me about protein foods?"

Fact Sheets allow the students the opportunity to share how much they know about a subject. You can give individual students or small groups a topic and ask them to come up with 10-20 facts (or answers if the topic is a question). Fact sheets can also be assigned as homework to encourage research.

To begin a fact sheet activity about comfort measures you might say, "List at least ten things you can do if a mother has a back labor. As you think of them, write them down so we can share our lists."

Listing, in which the students create a list based on the topic and then a second list of applicable responses to the topic, helps the students grasp the correlations when more than one answer is appropriate. As an example, the first list could be made as a list of signs and discomforts at a stage of labor. Then the students create a second list of ways to manage or handle the signs and discomforts.

To begin a listing activity about pregnancy discomforts you might say, "Tell me all the things pregnant women complain about. I'll write down your answers." After the list is complete you would continue, "Let's choose the five we think are the most common, and make a list of things we can do to reduce the amount of discomfort they cause."

Worksheets provide an easy way for students to evaluate their understanding of material. Worksheets can also provide an opportunity for personal reflection or assist in planning. Worksheets make it easy for students to learn at home between classes. Some worksheets are designed specifically for **personal reflection**. This gives the students the opportunity to consider how the new skills and knowledge they are gaining fits into their lives. A variety of worksheets are included in the student workbook and at the teacher web site.

To begin a nutrition worksheet activity you may say, "I've just passed out a menu planning worksheet. We can go over the instructions together, but I would like you to complete the worksheet as homework."

Mastery Activities

Because the goal of childbirth education is not simply to increase the expectant parents' knowledge, but to master skills necessary for coping with the stress of labor, you should provide opportunities for the students to practice using the information and skills they have gained. The following activities help the students move from knowledge of the concept to mastery of the skill.

Role Play allows the student to imagine themselves in a situation and gives them the opportunity to practice their response to that situation. Role plays do not need to be performed before the whole class, but can be worked out in small groups or by couples. Another effective use of role play is for the teacher to play a role and allow the students the opportunity to respond to that role.

To begin a role play activity you might say, "For the next few minutes all the expectant mom's are going to pretend to be in labor. I will give you a problem; for example, your back is sore. Moms will act out the problem, labor partners you quickly come up with a way to manage it and start acting out your solution.

Case Studies, review of an actual birth story, allow the students the chance to work through the events of labor and pick out important decision making points. When the case study is incorporated with some role playing, the students have the opportunity to experience the struggles of decision making in labor before they get there. Case studies are highly effective at promoting changes in attitudes.

To begin a case study activity you might say, "As you read this birth story, see if you there are places you might have made a different decision."

Problem Solving can be done in groups or as individuals to explore the possibilities and their effect on the labor as a whole. Case Studies can be used in problem solving, or the instructor can give a fictional scenario such as in a role play. The students then define the problem and establish a goal; determine the cause of the problem; seek solutions and then evaluate the alternatives and recommend a course of action.

To begin a problem solving activity about nutrition you might hand out menu cards and say, "You each have one day of meals for a pregnant woman. Is there anything that concerns you about you woman's meals? What could you do to improve her nutrition?"

Questioning, a lighter form of problem solving, can be used to stimulate thought and discussion on an issue. Questions posed by the teacher to the class can be a review of the material or can help assess the students understanding.

To begin a questioning activity about stages of labor you might say, "I am going to list some signs of progress in labor. You are going to tell me what stage of labor the mother is in."

Rehearsals of labor coping skills give the students the opportunity to respond to the demands of contractions and can incorporate problem solving as well. The student's ability to work as a team with her husband or labor partner improves as they work together to learn to respond to labor.

To begin a rehearsal you might say, "For the next half hour we will all behave as if labor is actually happening now."

Other Learning Aides

Video Presentations can offer students a view of what cannot be otherwise experienced. Actually seeing a woman in labor can help couples understand how the whole process works. Some videos offer graphical presentations of the birth process to help the students comprehend how it all works together. Videos are not good choices for material that can be understood through other means because a video in itself does not offer interaction or a way for students to work with the information they are receiving.

When a video is used, give the students a task such as determining what comfort measures are used or figuring out when the mother is at different stages of labor. Always give time for discussion and questions after a video presentation.

To begin a video presentation you might say, "We are going to watch a video of an actual birth now. As you watch the video, pay attention to the positions the mother uses so we can talk about them after the video is finished.

Games can be a fun way to help motivate students to master new material by engaging them in a friendly competition. Games can also help the students see just how much they have learned.

To begin a game about managing labor you might say, "We're going to have a little fun while we review what we have learned so far."

Interviews with doulas, nurses or families that have already given birth can give your students the opportunity to hear different sides of an issue and to experience the issues surrounding labor from another perspective.

To begin an interview you might say, "I would like to introduce you to one of our doulas who has agreed to answer questions you may have."

Field Trips to the birth center or local hospital can help students better understand the options available to them and increase their comfort level with the facility.

To begin a field trip you might say, "The birth pool is free tonight, so lets leave our things here while we take a few minutes to go see how big it really is."

Using the Activities in the Book

The activities in the Christian Childbirth Workbook and this teaching guide have been organized in units of study. These units follow the layout of the Christian Childbirth Handbook, and can fit easily into an eight week class format. However, this format will not fit every teaching need.

Some classes will benefit from splitting the units between all classes. In this style, each class would include an activity or two from several units. Examples may be review classes or informal Bible study classes.

Some classes will benefit from focusing on only a portion of the units. In this style, only the units relevant to the topic will be taught in class and others can be completed by families if they choose. Examples may be early pregnancy classes or breast feeding classes.

Some classes will benefit from selecting only the activities that will make the most impact in the shortest amount of time. In this style, specific pages, handouts and worksheets would be printed from the teacher web site and distributed to clients. Examples may be private classes or prenatal doula meetings.

Each activity has listed the estimated amount of time, materials you may choose to use and alternative teaching methods for the topic. As the class facilitator, you can choose which activities to include in a class, which to assign for homework and which to skip. The next chapter will help you begin the process of turning this collection of activities into your unique curriculum.

Chapter Six

Designing a Class

Part of your role as a childbirth educator is to take this collection of activities and present it in a way that offers your clients opportunities to master childbirth skills. You have the freedom to use the materials in this book and on the web site in whatever way God leads you. If you have been thinking about this book as a script you must follow, stop.

There is no childbirth curriculum that will meet every objective for every situation. The goals of a class must be flexible so you can meet the needs of each individual class or family. The topics chosen must change to accommodate experienced parents or unprepared teens. Activities must be varied to be appropriate for an all day class of single women or a several week course that includes siblings. Presentation styles must prevent boredom while ensuring continuity for the class. This means, the ability of your classes to meet the needs of your clients is dependent upon your ability to create one.

Designing Curriculum

The first step is to determine the purpose of your class. You may choose to teach a breast feeding or a parenting class. You may want to prepare families for home birth or for cesarean birth. You may provide VBAC classes, single parent classes, teen classes or refresher classes. You may find yourself offering several different types of classes. For each class, define your purpose.

Once you have defined the purpose of a class, you can begin to define the goals of your class. Your goal is not to teach childbirth classes. +That is the way you hope to achieve your goal. To discover what your goal is will require you to do much more reflection about yourself and your community.

The question is not if you have goals, but rather what those goals are. Carefully defining your goals for teaching will help you refine your class. It gives you the rule by which to measure your activities. Without clearly defined and written on paper goals for your class, you may frequently feel you have "left something out." Without clear goals you may spend time on unnecessary lecture or struggle with feeling like you constantly need to add more to your class.

The basic question to ask yourself as you define your goals is, "What do I want my students to be able to do after attending my class?" Some possible goals might include modifying health behaviors, making evidence-based decisions, or successfully use comfort techniques during labor.

Once you know your goal or goals, you can begin to set learning objectives. A learning objective is a specific piece of information or a skill your class needs to have to achieve the goal you have set. For example, if you set a goal that families will be successful at breast feeding, your learning objectives will include identifying proper latch; identifying proper position; managing common problems; and

23

assessing adequacy of breast milk supply. You may choose to teach more, but you cannot teach less and still meet your goal. Your list of objectives allows you to organize the content you wish to teach.

With your list of written objectives in hand, select the activities you would like to use to meet those objectives. As you select activities, consider how much time you have, what supplies are available to you and what other activities you would like to complete. You may need to select a faster activity for one objective to allow a longer activity for another objective. You may want to select two activities for more difficult material. Put your list of activities in the sequence you would like to present them to the class and you have your curriculum.

Be sure you understand any restraints you may have in your teaching location. You may be teaching in your home, a crisis pregnancy center, at your church, in a community center or at a hospital.

Be sure you understand the group you will be teaching. You may be working with teens, single women, married couples or whole families. Ensure you have the right material and warm-up activities for each unique class group.

The final step is evaluation of each class after you have taught it. Reflect on the activities chosen and their success with the class. Make adjustments as necessary to ensure your classes successfully achieve your goals.

Teaching Secrets

The success of your classes depends on you. However, there are a few secrets you can learn to help achieve success more frequently.

Estimate how much time each activity will take, and write it as a class schedule. Keep that schedule nearby, and look at a clock every so often to be sure you are on target for completing all the material within the time-frame allotted.

Always plan a few extra activities in case the class moves through material faster than you anticipated. Having a game or labor rehearsal available gives your students extra time to master skills and gives you additional opportunity to assess the class learning.

Gather your materials the day before you plan to teach. If you are missing materials, you will still have time to plan a different activity to meet the learning objective.

Try not to teach from detailed notes. This prevents you from making eye contact with the class and increases the amount of time it takes to teach. Instead, make an outline with headings for each topic you want to cover or the name of an activity.

Assigning readings or homework assignments increases the amount of material you are able to cover as a class, promotes self learning among your students and improves in-class interaction. However, not every class will be inclined to complete homework.

Try to end your class with an activity that allows you to assess if your students have learned the day's material. If they appear to be experiencing difficulty, you can use another activity to help re-teach. If necessary, you can do a review exercise as a warm-up for the next class.

Look over your class schedule from the standpoint of your students. Make a list, in chronological order, of what a student is doing during your class. Are the activities alternated to keep the class interesting, or are you planning to have students listening to a lecture and watching a video during the entire class?

Additional Materials

There are additional materials you can use as you design your course on the teaching web site. This is a private site, and you will need to use the following information to get in:

http://www.birthingnaturally.net/teaching/index.html

Log in with the User Name: teacher

Log in with the Password: workbook

While checking out the materials, be sure to submit your contact information to the teacher list so families can find your services.

It is time to start designing your class. Begin by thinking about all the factors that will affect how you should design your class. Complete the sentences in step one before moving on to step two. Use additional paper if necessary. Answer the questions for step three, then move on to the next page..

Step One: Class Purpose

The purpose defines the reason for the class. This will usually be to fill a need you see in your community. Your class purpose is also determined by the unique calling God has placed on your life.

I want to teach Christian childbirth classes because...

The biggest needs I see for expectant families in my community are...

My purpose as a childbirth educator is...

Step Two: Class Goals and Learning Objectives

Your goals are the way you hope to fulfill the purpose identified during step one. Defining your class goals allows you to determine which activities are valuable to fulfilling your classes purpose. This helps avoid wasted time.

After my classes, I expect my students to...

The skills my students need to accomplish this are...

If my students are to achieve the class goals, my classes must cover...

For my students to understand the material, I should cover the information in this order...

Step Three: Learning Activities

The learning activities are the things you do in your class to meet your goals and objectives so you can fulfill your purpose. The activities chosen will depend on many factors including the space and time available to you, your client background and the materials you can access for class.

Teaching Location Questions:

Where will you be teaching your classes?

What is the size of the room?

What furniture is available to you?

How much open floor space do you have?

How much time is available for set up and clean up?

How much time is available for teaching in each class?

Client Information:

How many clients do you expect in the class?

How many couples will attend?

How many single women will attend?

How many families with children will attend?

Will your clients know each other before attending your class?

How much experience with childbirth will your clients have before attending your class?

What special needs will your clients have while attending your class?

Learning Activities

Because of my teaching location and client background, I want to select learning activities that...

Because of my teaching location and client background, I want to avoid learning activities that..

Materials I would like to acquire to facilitate learning activities are...

Designing your Curriculum

To your curriculum, you will need to combine the information about your learning goals and objectives with the information about your learning activities. To begin, outline the topics you need to cover to meet your goals. This does not need to be perfect, just your first guess. Your classes will evolve as you teach them.

Your second step is to determine what activities you would like to use for each topic. Estimate the amount of time each activity will take (more, less or the same as the estimated time given for the activity). Review your list for any areas you might have missed and add activities for those units. Add together the estimated activity times to see the total amount of teaching time you will need.

Think about how you want to break up that total teaching time to fit the time you have available at your teaching location. Does it fit neatly into four, six or eight weeks with two hours of class time? Can it realistically be completed in one day with regular breaks? Do not forget to add any time you may need for snacks and fellowship.

If your activities do not fill the time you allotted for the classes you have two choices. You can change the class scheduled to shorter or fewer sessions, or you can add additional activities.

If your activities will take more time than you allotted for the classes, you have two choices. You can change the class schedule to either longer or more sessions, or you can remove some activities.

With your schedule breakdown determined and the activities chosen, organize the activities into weeks or sessions. Think about how the students will build their understanding and place activities for learning more basic skills before the more advanced skills.

Finally, choose one activity as your backup for each week or session. You do not need to complete this activity, but have it ready in case the class moves through the material faster than you anticipated.

You can make copies of the table on the next page to help plan your overall curriculum. Use copies of the class planning form on page 28 to write out the full plan for each week or session of your class. Think about the order of the activities in each session and what materials you will need to complete those activities. Remember, you can and will make changes to your class plan as you become more experienced.

Class Evaluation

After each class, spend some time evaluating the experience. This will help you identify activities to change, information you should add and places where your knowledge should increase. The following questions will help you evaluate your class.

Did you leave enough time to complete each activity or extra time without an activity planned?

Did you misjudge how much time each activity would take, or was time estimation for one activity wrong?

Did you give enough instruction, or too much instruction before beginning the activity?

Is there another activity that you would like to try for the next series of classes?

Did the activities help the class master the class objectives?

Did you correctly anticipate the previous knowledge about the concepts discussed?

Did the material move too quickly or too slowly?

Does the class need additional teaching before moving on?

Were questions and activities completed appropriately?

Did the questions the class asked demonstrate an understanding of the material?

Did the class enjoy the activities chosen?

Did the class participate willingly?

Was the conversation productive?

Did you have enough materials for the activities chosen?

Were you comfortable with the information you were teaching?

What questions arose that you were unable to answer?

What additional research would you like to do before teaching this class again?

Class Planning Outline

Copy as needed, or print this document from the teaching web site.

Topic	Activity	Teaching Time	Week or Session

Class Planning Outline

Copy as needed, or print this document from the teaching web site.

Time	Topic	Learner Objectives	Teaching Materials

Sample Class Planning Outline

Use this sample to help you understand how to complete a planning outline.

Time	Topic	Learner Objectives	Teaching Materials
15 min.	Welcome	The learner will feel welcome in the class and willing to participate in activities. • Have participants write down three things they want to learn. • Volunteers will organize the items into categories as we learn each person's name and the three things they want to learn.	Post it notes Markers
15 min.	Spiritual significance of Pregnancy	The learner will be able to list three reasons pregnancy is a spiritually significant event. • Have volunteer read the passage. • Discuss the questions, writing key points on dry erase board.	Page 12 of workbook Bibles Dry erase board
10 min.	Changes in mom and baby	The learner will be able to describe three common pregnancy complaints and list ways to help relieve them. • Begin by explaining the hormonal changes in pregnancy. • Ask for ideas of ways to manage common discomforts.	Hormonal Changes Flier Dry erase board

Part Two

Teaching Activities

Overview

This first unit sets the stage for families to understand the significance of the decisions they make regarding pregnancy and childbirth. It presents a framework for determining how to set priorities while addressing lifestyle issues that may affect pregnancy outcomes.

Nutrition, exercise, normal process of pregnancy and managing discomforts of pregnancy are all included in this first unit because they are inter-related. Helping families understand this truth not only improves their attitude and acceptance of pregnancy and their new baby, but also improves their chances of having a normal labor.

This information is presented through the Christian concept of stewardship; using the gifts God has given you to serve his purposes. It is as important to ensure you are making appropriate decisions for the physical needs of your body and your baby as it is to ensure you are making appropriate decisions with how you spend your money, time and other resources.

Unit Goals

After finishing the material in this unit, your students should be able to:

• Perform specific pregnancy exercises
• Plan healthy menus for their family
• Identify ways to mange pregnancy discomforts
• Recognize the significance of decisions they make

Suggested Reading

Christian Childbirth Handbook

What is Christian Childbirth?
Healthy Pregnancy

40 Weeks

Part One: Healthy Pregnancy

Birthing Naturally Web site

Pregnancy Exercise
Pregnancy Nutrition

Sample Schedule

Time	Activity	Workbook Page
15 Minutes	Eternal Significance	12
10 Minutes	Changes in Mother and Baby	13-14
30 Minutes	Pregnancy Exercises	15-17
30 Minutes	Pregnancy Nutrition	18-20
25 Minutes	Stewardship	21-22

Workbook Page 11

Overview

This pregnancy is a gift from God. Right now you are growing and caring for one of God's children. You are accountable to God for how you use the resources he has given you to care for this child. You are also accountable to God for the decisions you make which affect this child while in your care. How you care for the things God has given you is stewardship.

To help you make the best decisions for the health of your child, you will need to educate yourself about how to keep both mother and baby healthy. Eating a nutritious diet is one of the best ways to maintain good health. Keeping your body active not only helps you feel more comfortable and energetic, but also prepares your body for labor.

You will also find you have options for how to handle the normal discomforts of pregnancy. Understanding the options available will help you be a good steward of this pregnancy.

Discussion Points

✓ How you treat your body is a matter of stewardship. Make the best use of the resources God has given you to keep yourself and your baby healthy.

✓ The quality of your diet will have a significant impact on your health.

✓ In general, whole foods served as close to their natural state as possible will be the best options for optimal health.

✓ American College of Obstetricians and Gynecologists (ACOG) recommends that pregnant women exercise daily, citing that exercise during pregnancy is linked to healthier pregnancies and fewer problems in labor.

✓ Many pregnancy discomforts can be handled by making changes in diet and exercise habits.

Self-Study

✒ Follow the principles of good nutrition and exercise for one week. How does your body feel different? What was difficult about this experience? What was enjoyable about this experience?

✒ Look through different directions God has given about eating. Adam and Eve (Genesis 2:16), Noah (Genesis 9:3) and Moses (Leviticus 11:3-4) were all given different guidelines. Explore what else the Bible has to say about food. In what ways does what you believe about God affect the way you eat?

✒ Keep a food journal for one to three days. Enter this information into a free online nutrition analysis program. How does your nutrition stack up?

Unit One
Stewardship

Scripture Checklist
- ❑ Matthew 25:14-30
- ❑ Luke 12:47-48
- ❑ 1 Corinthians 6:19-20
- ❑ Jeremiah 10:23
- ❑ 2 Corinthians 5:15
- ❑ Psalm 24:1
- ❑ Luke 16:10
- ❑ 1 Corinthians 4:2
- ❑ Galatians 6:9
- ❑ Matthew 6:19-20
- ❑ Psalm 193:14
- ❑
- ❑
- ❑
- ❑

Suggested Readings
Christian Childbirth Handbook

What is Christian Childbirth?
Healthy Pregnancy

40 Weeks

Part One: Healthy Pregnancy

Birthing Naturally Web site

Pregnancy Exercise
Pregnancy Nutrition

11

33

Title: **What is Eternally Significant About Pregnancy?**

Page: 12

Activity: Discussion

Purpose: Set the stage for pregnancy as a stewardship issue. Provide opportunity for families to evaluate their current priorities.

Time: 10-15 minutes

Directions: Begin by having class members spend a few minutes writing down their response to the question, "What is Eternally Significant About Pregnancy?" Ask group members to share their responses.

Direct the class attention to the potential for spiritual growth during pregnancy. Ask class members to share ideas of how to foster this growth.

Finally, ask the class to write decisions they have made about this pregnancy during the last week or month. Ask them to consider what these decisions reveal about their heart and priorities. Have they been setting their priorities in search of the eternally significant?

Facilitating: Giving the class time to think and write down their answers will help improve participation in a discussion.

If you write answers on a large sheet of paper or dry erase board you will improve participation in the discussion.

If the class is very large (more than 12 people), ask them to split into two or three smaller groups for discussion during this exercise.

Materials: Pens
Bibles

Scripture: Matthew 6:19-20
Do not store up for yourselves treasures on earth, where moth and rust destroy, and where thieves break in and steal. But store up for yourselves treasures in heaven, where moth and rust do not destroy, and where thieves do not break in and steal.

Treasure you can store in heaven is the eternally significant things in life. Many of the things we focus on with pregnancy and childbirth, such as weight gain or where you give birth are not eternally significant. However, these issues may be significant in as far as decisions you make can reveal the condition of your heart.

Whether your heart is serving God or serving self is eternally significant. Consider the actions you take and decisions you make. Are these decisions made from a heart of fear, or a heart desiring to serve God?

<table>
<tr>
<td>

Unit One
Stewardship
My Thoughts...

</td>
<td>

What is eternally significant about pregnancy?

Matthew 6:19-20 calls us to seek out that which is eternally significant. The question is, "What exactly is eternally significant about pregnancy?"

What are some ways you can use this time of pregnancy to:
Build your faith?

Give glory to God?

Mature spiritually?

Witness to those around you?

This unit focuses on the eternal significance of the decisions you make. Though specific decisions may not be significant in themselves, the process you use to make the decision can reveal where your heart is. Are you making decisions as a good steward of what God has given you, or are you making decisions to serve yourself. It all comes down to stewardship. Did you do your best with what God put in your care?

Discussion Question:
Reflecting on the decisions you have already made for this pregnancy, what is revealed about your heart by the way you make decisions?

</td>
</tr>
</table>

12

Title:	**Changes in Mother**
Page:	13
Activity:	Lecture with Discussion
Purpose:	Identify physical changes within the mother, and what she can do to manage any discomfort from those changes.
Time:	5-10 minutes
Directions:	Draw a chart to represent the normal hormonal changes in women during pregnancy. Point out the high levels of estrogen and progesterone. Explain the way high progesterone levels affect the body system by system.

While discussing changes, ask the class for ideas of ways to manage the discomfort. Be sure to give any answers they were unable to identify on their own. |
| Facilitating: | Be sure you have a good understanding of the hormones of pregnancy before beginning this topic to prevent confusion. 40 Weeks Devotional Guide gives an overview of the hormonal changes if you need a description.

Use the new understanding of the causes of pregnancy discomforts as a way to encourage good nutrition and exercise habits in the next sections. To stimulate discussion you might ask, "What might affect the difference in how these changes affect different women?" |
| Materials: | Dry erase board or large paper
Appropriate markers
Chart of pregnancy hormone levels |
| Scripture: | Genesis 2

God had a purpose for female fertility before the fall. It was not a curse nor an afterthought.

At this point you may choose to do the activity on Workbook page 25 to help families understand that pregnancy and birth were part of God's original perfect creation. |

Changes in Mother

Pregnancy changes the mother's circulating levels of progesterone and estrogen which is essential to maintain a pregnancy. However, the increased progesterone levels also cause some changes in the mother's body. List some things you can do to minimize the discomforts caused by these changes.

Digestion
Your digestive system is relaxed by progesterone. This can make digestion sluggish causing heartburn and constipation.

Circulation
Your circulatory system is also made of smooth muscle and so is relaxed by progesterone. Your body increases the amount of circulating blood during pregnancy. Your heart pumps more blood, faster than it did before you were pregnant. You may feel dizzy in extreme heat or when you stand up fast. Your body may feel puffy due to the increased circulation.

Breasts
Progesterone and estrogen stimulate your mammary glands to mature and prepare to produce milk. This may cause tenderness and sensitivity as well as an increase in breast size.

Respiration
Progesterone also causes your lung capacity to increase to meet the increased need for oxygen and to remove carbon dioxide. You may notice you breathe faster and your rib cage has expanded.

13

Title: **Changes in Baby**

Page: 14

Activity: Lecture

Purpose: Identify the detailed process of development and ways to facilitate normal growth for the rest of the pregnancy.

Time: No more than 5 minutes

Directions: Point out the page in the workbook to your families. Invite them to glance over the process of development.

Ask them to find the point in development that matches where they are in their pregnancy and read what is and will be happening to their baby in the next few weeks. Display a fetal growth chart to help families visualize the development of their baby.

Point out that babies grow and develop right up to the moment of birth, and that development of body systems continues even after birth. The brain and nervous system, the musculature and the digestive system go through times of tremendous development during the first two years.

Facilitating: Use the new understanding about what is developing in their baby to encourage families to pay better attention to their nutrition.

Families interested in the mysteries of God may enjoy studying the way pregnancy milestones line up with the timing of Jewish feasts. This information can be found in the video A Child is Born available from Zola Levitt Ministries. Summaries of this teaching are found in 40 Weeks Devotional Guide to Pregnancy.

More detailed decsriptions of the changes in late pregnancy can be found in 40 Weeks Devotionl Guide to Pregnancy.

Materials: Fetal development chart
Fetal development video
A Child is Born video

Scripture: Psalm 193:14
I praise you because I am fearfully and wonderfully made;
your works are wonderful,
I know that full well.

Your baby was not created by accident. God has created this specific child to meet a need for his plan. Your child is being designed with the gifts and talents needed to become the person God wants her to be. Although her personality may mature as she grows, her temperament has already been set.

Unit One
Stewardship
My Thoughts...

Changes in Baby

Your baby begins growing and forming from the moment of conception. The internal organs are formed by the 10th week of pregnancy, however most systems will continue to mature as your baby grows. Here are some highlights of your baby's development. (Weeks are given in gestational time, about two weeks behind your pregnancy week.)

Day 1:   Fertilization, the sperm and egg meet and begin to make your baby.

Day 10:   Your baby implants in the uterine wall.

Week 2:   The bag of waters forms around your baby. The placenta begins to form and grow to bring food, water and oxygen to your baby.

Week 3:   Lung buds, heart and central nervous system begin to form.

Week 4:   Face and internal organs begin to develop. Circulation begins.

Week 5:   External ears, eyes, nose, arm and leg buds begin to develop. Brain and spinal cord are well developed. Baby's blood vessels are working.

Week 6:   Testes or Ovaries develop. Vertebrae are laid down, and there is rapid brain growth. Only 1/4 inch long.

Week 7:   Nasal openings, fingers and toes, muscle fibers begin to develop.

Week 8:   Human facial features well developed. Teeth form. Penis appears.

Week 9:   Mini human look. Major blood vessels almost formed. Just over one inch long.

At the End of:

3 Months: Baby has primitive hair follicles and finger nails. Baby can make fists, open mouth, squint face and is about 3 inches long.

4 Months: Baby has a mini adult brain. Her eyebrows and lashes are growing. The heartbeat is audible with a stethoscope. Baby is 8 ½ inches long.

5 Months: The midpoint of your pregnancy, you have probably felt the baby move. Baby has hair on his head and is skinny at 12 inches and only 1 pound. Fat is beginning to be deposited under his skin.

6 Months: Baby's skin has a protective cover called vernix. Baby's eyes open and will soon be sensitive to light. The ears can hear. Your baby has finger and foot prints. Baby is around 14 inches long, 2 pounds.

7 Months: Taste buds have developed, and the organs are developed well enough for him to survive. 16 inches long and 3 ½ pounds.

8 Months: Her brain is growing rapidly, and so is her body. She is putting on fat and may weigh 5 pounds and be 18 inches long.

9 Months: He is putting on fat as he waits to be born, your baby is around 7 pounds and 20 inches long. He has about an inch of hair on his head and his skin is red.

14

Title:	**Pregnancy Exercises**
Page:	15
Type:	Listing
Purpose:	List the benefits of different types of exercise.
Time:	10 minutes
Directions:	Begin by asking the families to share how they work exercise into their daily lives.
	Have families list the specific benefits of exercise during pregnancy, including ways exercise helps overcome the normal discomforts from the changes of pregnancy.
	Briefly share the three types of exercise and specific benefits. Encourage families to share their favorite exercise for each category.
	Ask families to quickly write out a daily or weekly exercise schedule they could use to improve their fitness during this pregnancy. If time allows, have families share their ideas.
Facilitating:	Benefits of pregnancy exercise are explained in The Christian Childbirth Handbook and 40 Weeks Devotional Guide to Pregnancy.
	Familiarize yourself with the ACOG (or your national obstetrical organization's) guidelines for pregnancy exercise so you are prepared to answer questions. A copy of the ACOG guidelines is available at the Birthing Naturally web site.
Materials:	ACOG guidelines for Exercise
Scripture:	1 Corinthians 4:2 Now it is required that those who have been given a trust must prove faithful.
	It is well known that exercise in pregnancy improves the health of the mother and the baby. In general it is also able to have a positive effect in labor. As a steward of health, exercise should be a priority. Yet exercise is often not a high enough priority during pregnancy.
	Why does exercise frequently end up at the bottom of priority lists? What can be done to improve faithfulness with exercise.

Pregnancy Exercises

Pregnancy Exercise

List the reasons to exercise during pregnancy.

Types of Exercise

List your favorite exercises from each type.

Strength

Flexibility

Cardiovascular

Your Exercise Schedule:

Think about your daily schedule. Are there days you have more or less time for activity? Are there ways you can adjust your schedule to increase the amount of activity? Write out a sample exercise schedule here:

Monday

Tuesday

Wednesday

Thursday

Friday

Saturday

Sunday

Unit One
Stewardship
My Thoughts...

15

Title:	**The Kegel Muscle**
Page:	16
Type:	Guided Discovery
Purpose:	Improve adherence to recommended Kegel practice schedule.
Time:	10 minutes
Directions:	Have families label the diagram of the pelvic structures. Discuss the purpose of the Kegel muscle and the added strain on this muscle during pregnancy.
	Explain the process of learning to do a Kegel exercise; let the women practice as you explain how.
	Share the method of relaxing the Kegel muscle, and how this will benefit the pushing stage of labor.
	Ask families to share ways they can be reminded to Kegel every day.
Facilitating:	This exercise takes practice, allow a few minutes at the beginning or ending of class each week to introduce the next step.
	This exercise may make some families uncomfortable. Be confident and present the diagram in a matter-of-fact manner. Your comfort will help families be more comfortable.
	You can distribute Kegel stickers to help your families remember to practice this exercise. Templates for stickers are on the teacher web site.
Materials:	Model Pelvis Kegel Stickers

Workbook Page 16

My Thoughts...

The Kegel Muscle

Label the pelvic structures.

Bladder

Cervix

Coccyx

Pelvic Floor (Kegel) Muscle

Rectum

Uterus

Vagina

Why do Kegel exercises?

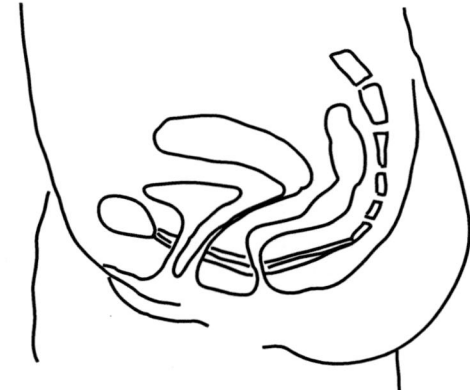

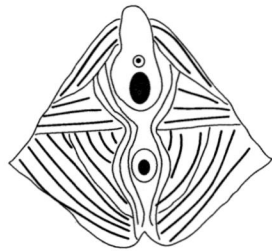

How to do it

To begin, try to isolate the pelvic floor by contracting it as if you were trying to stop the flow of urine. Do not worry at first about letting go of the contraction; just let it relax on its own. As you get stronger you will learn how to let go of the contraction.

Begin building the strength of the muscle by holding the contraction for 1 second, then 2 seconds and eventually up to 3 seconds.

When you are strong enough to hold the contraction for 3 seconds, increase your control of the muscle by contracting a little, then a little more, then all the way. Learn to contract the muscle in increments before you begin to learn to relax the muscle in increments.

The last step is to learn to relax, or bulge the muscle. This is the same movement you use to release the flow of urine. After contracting the muscle, bulge it out (if you have difficultly determining if the muscle is bulged, put your hand along the perineum. You should feel it bulge out as you relax the Kegel muscle)

16

Title:	**Pelvic Tilt & Squatting**
Page:	17
Type:	Guided Discovery
Purpose:	Improve adherence to recommended exercise regime.
Time:	10 minutes
Directions:	Discuss the benefits of performing pelvic tilt exercises.
	Demonstrate pelvic tilting, then have mothers practice the exercise. Ask the mothers how it feels and when they think they might like to practice this exercise every day.
	Discuss the benefits of performing squat exercises.
	Demonstrate squatting, then have mothers practice the exercise. Ask the mothers how squatting feels and when they think they might like to practice this exercise every day.
	Explain the benefits of sitting cross-legged. Ask families to sit cross-legged on the floor during classes.
	Include additional exercises as appropriate.
Facilitating:	Providing exercise mats is not necessary, but some couples will feel more comfortable if they are available. You can recommend they bring them to class if they would like them.
	If a family is not performing an exercise correctly, point out what they are doing right first, then suggest they make necessary changes to get the most benefit from the exercise.
	If you do not have couples practice the exercises in class, they probably will not do them at home.
Materials:	Open space Exercise Mats

Pelvic Tilt

Why Pelvic Tilt?

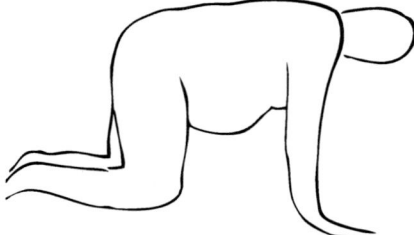

How to do it

While on hands and knees, tilt your pelvis under by contracting deep abdominal muscles. While you are learning, try to pay close attention to the abdominal contraction. This will prevent you from trying to tilt your pelvis by arching your back. When it is done properly, the movement is very small and your back should stay relatively flat.

Squatting

Why Squat?

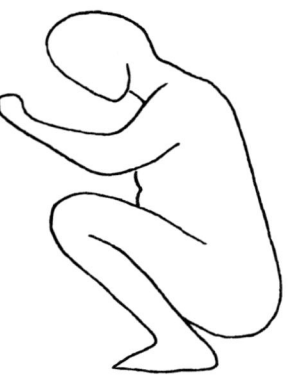

How to do it

Keeping your feet firmly planted on the floor, lower your upper body into a slight bend; lower your bottom to the floor by bending your knees and hips.

If you find it is difficult to keep your balance, stand in front of a table, counter, heavy chair or another person, and hold on while you lower your body.

17

Title:	**Pregnancy Nutrition**
Page:	18
Type:	List Making
Purpose:	Identify changes in diet that could benefit pregnancy.
Time:	10 minutes

Directions: Begin by sharing the various recommendations for adequate nutrition during pregnancy. Have families list the reasons for eating each nutrient. Ask families to recall what they have eaten in the previous 24 hours and compare their diet to the recommendations.

Because each family is unique, ask them to share any concerns they may have about their diet, and how they may be able to address those concerns. If the group is willing, other members of the class may be able to provide suggestions as well.

Facilitating: Families may miscalculate the number of servings they eat if they are not familiar with the standard servings sizes. Be sure to have a chart handy or be familiar enough with the sizes to explain.

Using sample meal cards rather than the mother's personal diet allows families to develop nutritional evaluation skills without embarrassing anyone.

Be familiar with Dr. Tom Brewer's teachings about pregnancy nutrition to answer questions.

Differences in serving recommendations occur because countries approach the recommendations differently. For example, the USA uses the same recommendations for all adults adding an additional dairy for pregnancy; so more active adults would eat more servings. Other countries provide separate recommendations for different population groups.

Materials: Serving-size Chart
Meal Cards

Scripture: 1 Corinthians 6:19-20
Do you not know that your body is a temple of the Holy Spirit, who is in you, whom you have received from God? You are not your own; you were bought at a price. Therefore honor God with your body.

Though this passage is written with respect to sexual immorality, it is applicable to all the ways we treat our body. How can what you eat honor God with your body?

Workbook Page 18

Unit One
Stewardship
My Thoughts...

Pregnancy Nutrition

Various Recommendations for Adequate Nutrition in Pregnancy

Food Group	Dr. Brewer	USA	Canada	Australia	UK
Protein	4	2-3	2	1.5	Moderate
Dairy	4	2	2	2	2-3
Fruits and Vegetables	5	5-9	7-8	9-10	5
Grains	4	6-11	6-7	4-6	1/3 of diet
Pregnancy Specific	NA	1 additional dairy serving	Add 2-3 servings of any group	NA	NA

Why do you need each type of nutrient?

Protein:

Carbohydrates:

Fat:

Discussion Questions:
What concerns do you have about the way you eat?
What drives your decisions about what to eat?

18

Title: **Make it Nutrient Dense**

Page: 19

Type: List Making

Purpose: Create a list of usable ideas to ensure adequate protein intake.

Time: 5 minutes

Directions: Introduce the worksheet to the families. Ask them to list three to five suggestions they would enjoy using for each category. They should write their answers on this sheet.

Give families three or four minutes to think about the question and write in their answers. Ask families to share one of their favorite nutrient dense foods with the class.

Facilitating: If you have time and resources, you may have families calculate their total grams of protein within the previous 24 hours for comparison to the 75 gram minimum standard set by Dr. Brewer.

An alternate presentation is to use the Menu Planning Worksheet available on the teaching web site. Families could then complete the meal planning exercise on page 20 at home.

If you choose to provide a snack for class, use the snack as a sample of a nutrient dense food.

The Birthing Naturally web site offers a cookbook with recipes rated for good pregnancy nutrition to help families learn how to compare recipes.

If families need help thinking of add-in ideas, suggest they think about ways to use eggs and cheese. Do they enjoy any nuts or seeds? What types of beans do they like to eat?

Materials: Meal Cards
Menu Planning Worksheet

Workbook Page 19

Make it Nutrient Dense

What can you add to make these foods more nutrient dense?
List your favorite food additions for each category.

Add to Salads:

Add to Sandwiches:

Add to Soups:

Add to Baked Goods:

List your favorite nutrient dense snacks.

List your favorite nutrient dense side dishes.

List your favorite nutrient dense toppings.

Quick Meal Ideas

Which of these quick meal ideas fit into your lifestyle?
- Bowl of Cereal, toast with peanut butter, glass of milk
- Cottage cheese with fruit
- Yogurt with fruit and granola
- Grilled cheese sandwich, salad or fresh vegetables
- Slice of cheese, English muffin or toast, piece of fruit
- Tuna sandwich, fruit
- Mixed nuts, piece of cheese, glass of juice
- Dry cereal with yogurt
- Peanut Butter and Jelly sandwich, fresh vegetables
- Instant soup or can of soup
- Popcorn, piece of cheese, piece of fruit

Add more ideas:

My Thoughts...

19

Title: **Meal Planning**

Page: 20

Type: Worksheet

Purpose: Understand that excellent pregnancy nutrition is possible with any income and schedule.

Time: 15 minutes

Directions: Provide families with a copy of the meal planning worksheet. Ask them to think about the foods they most enjoy eating and how they might fit into a pregnancy diet.

Have families prepare three days of menus following the standards for pregnancy nutrition.

Ask families to share what was easiest and most difficult about planning their menu.

Facilitating: Providing a sample menu may help your families understand what a daily meal menu can look like. Sample menus are available at the Birthing Naturally Web site.

Asking families to share their favorite foods and how they fit into pregnancy nutrition before completing the meal planning worksheet will give them ideas of foods to use.

Working in small groups may make it easier for some families to understand the meal planning process.

Beginning with dinner and working backwards through the daily meals can help. Using snacks to fill in gaps also makes the process easier. Have families modify the worksheet to fit their eating patterns. If they do not eat an evening snack, they do not need to list one.

Materials: Sample Menus

Scripture: Luke 16:10
Whoever can be trusted with very little can also be trusted with much, and whoever is dishonest with very little will also be dishonest with much.

What you eat may seem like such a small thing. But it has more effect on your health than nearly any other decision you make. How does knowing this change your perceptions of the importance of nutrition as a stewardship issue?

Unit One
Stewardship
My Thoughts...

Meal Planning
Plan three days of meals following the dietary recommendations.

	Day One	Day Two	Day Three
Breakfast			
Morning Snack			
Lunch			
Afternoon Snack			
Dinner			
Evening Snack			

Pointers:
Think outside the dinner plate. Six smaller meals may work better for you than 3 large meals.

Use the foods you know you like. You do not have to eat chicken if you hate it.

Double a recipe and use the leftovers for a lunch or freeze them for a quick dinner later in the month.

Eggs are not just a breakfast food. Keep deviled or hard boiled eggs for quick snacks.

Discussion Question:
How easy or difficult was it to create a nutritious menu?

20

Title: **Stewardship of Pregnancy**

Page: 21

Type: Worksheet

Purpose: Recognize the changes that need to be made during pregnancy and early parenting as well as changes which can be made to make life easier.

Time: 15 minutes

Directions: Ensure each family has a copy of the "Stewardship Wheel."

                Ask families to share the biggest challenges they have experienced since becoming pregnant.

                Ask families to share any big challenges they expect to have after their baby is born.

                Have families work individually to complete the worksheet, filling in changes they have already made or will need to make due to pregnancy.

                Have each family select one change to share with the group. Ask them to share why they felt that change was necessary.

Facilitating: Families may feel frustrated with this exercise at first, especially if this is their first baby. Be sure to be patient and give them the full amount of time to work. Quiet time with their thoughts or spouse will allow them to think through the question and provide them with good answers.

                Many families are not aware of the enormity of some challenges they will face. Your job is not to convince them your list of potential challenges is better than their list. Trust the Holy Spirit to prompt them and grow them at the pace that is right for them. However, if a family is not able to think of any challenge, suggest one or two to get them started.

Scripture: 2 Corinthians 5:15
                And he died for all, that those who live should no longer live for themselves but for him who died for them and was raised again.

                In what ways does being a Christian affect the way you handle the changes that come with pregnancy and a new baby?

My Thoughts...

Stewardship of Pregnancy

Your pregnancy and your baby will change your life in many ways. Some changes you may have expected, others may have come as a surprise to you. Take a few minutes to consider ways your life has changed since becoming pregnant, and the ways it will change after your baby is born. List the changes in the appropriate area of the diagram below. Consider how these changes affect your other responsibilities, and what you can do to prepare for them.

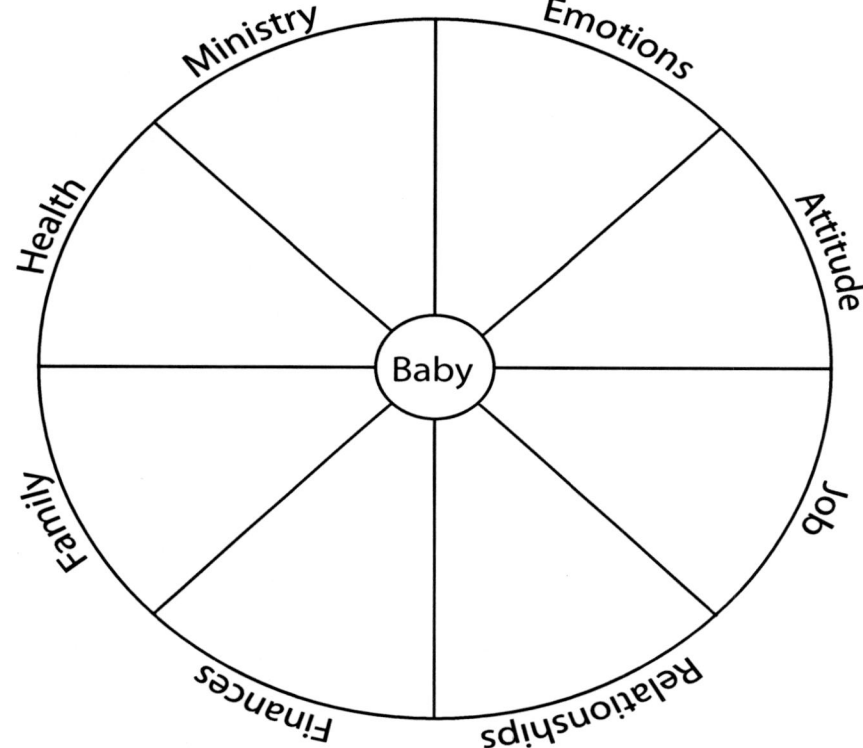

Discussion Question:
What possible changes have you anticipated?
How can you be prepared for those changes?

21

Title: **10 Easy Changes I Can Make**

Page: 22

Type: Worksheet

Purpose: Identify ways to be a good steward during pregnancy.

Time: 10 minutes

Directions: Remind the families of all the topics explored during this unit. Highlight any special points that came out.

Remind the families they have already identified several things they can do to help ensure a healthy pregnancy.

Ask families to make a list of ten easy things they can begin doing today to be a good steward of this pregnancy.

Facilitating: This is not supposed to be a list of general items like "eat better." It should be a very family-specific list of things to do. Instead of saying "eat better," a family may write "keep fresh vegetables in the house for snacks."

Families may feel the list should be of "important" or "big" items. Remind them that something as simple as getting adequate sleep helps improve health during pregnancy, so "go to bed by eleven each night" would be significant enough to make a difference.

Scripture: Jeremiah 10:23
I know, O LORD, that a man's life is not his own;
it is not for man to direct his steps.

If you have trouble coming up with things you can do, spend some time in prayer to let God direct the changes you make.

Unit One
Stewardship

My Thoughts...

10 Easy Changes I Can Make

Please list 10 specific things you can do in your everyday life to improve your health during this pregnancy. Instead of saying "eat healthy," say what you will do such as keep cut vegetables in the refrigerator.

1.

2.

3.

4.

5.

6.

7.

8.

9.

10.

22

Title: **Understanding My Body**

Page: 23

Type: Worksheet

Purpose: Identify personal needs for relaxation.

Time: Homework

Directions: Explain to families that God has created each person as a unique individual. No two women will have the same labor. Given the same circumstances, no two women will respond to labor the same way. This means how you manage labor will need to fit how you are uniquely created.

               Present the worksheet to families. Remind them that to be effective, comfort measures should be tailored to individual needs. Encourage them to fill this form out before the next class.

Facilitating: Return to this form during the second class to allow families a chance to discover how each woman is different in her needs for coping with pain.

               Some families may benefit from having the mother and her labor partner complete the worksheet for themselves to identify natural differences in the way they manage discomfort. Other families may benefit from having both the mother and labor partner fill it out for the mother to identify miscommunication about the mother's needs.

Understanding My Body

This worksheet is designed to help you prepare for the upcoming birth by identifying the way your body handles stress and pain. You should think about all sources of stress or discomfort, physical and emotional. Think of recent situations you have been in and consider how you responded to those situations.

I know I am feeling tense or stressed when my body…

My body reacts to tension by…

To remain clam while stressed I...

To cope with pain, I prefer…

Be Alone	or	Be With People
Keep Myself Busy	or	Tune Into Myself
Distract My Thoughts	or	Explore My Thoughts
Be Quiet	or	Talk With Someone
To be Touched	or	Not to Be Touched
Have Someone Help	or	Work it Out Alone

What has been your experience with using the following stress and pain coping techniques?

• Slow Deep Breathing

• Massage

• Visualization or Meditation on Scripture

• Vocalization

• Progressive Relaxation

• Using a Focus Point

• Prayer

Unit One
Stewardship
My Thoughts...

Circle your stress responses:

Head
Tension Headache
Tired Eyes
Grinding Teeth
Clenching Jaw
Ringing in Ears

Neck
Muscle Tightness
Decreased Range of Motion

Shoulders/Arms
Muscle Tightness
Trembling Hands
Gripping Fists
Biting Nails

Chest
Heart rate increasing
Heart pounding
Difficulty catching breath

Stomach
"Butterflies" in Stomach
Nausea

Back
Muscle Tightness
Sore Back
Bad Posture

Skin
Sweating
Clammy Skin
Itching/Scratching

Legs/Feet
Bouncing Legs
Trembling Feet
Sore or Achy Feet
Muscle Tension

Mental Processes
Speech Difficulties
Inability to Focus

23

Workbook Page 24 contains two devotional thoughts families can read.

Notes on **Scripture Checklist** from page 11

We begin with the parable of the talents (**Matthew 25:14-30; Luke 12:47-48**), a story about managing well the things God has given you. While the stewards in the story have been entrusted with gold coins, the concept of being a good steward is applicable to all parts of your life. You make choices every day from what to eat, when to sleep, how to exercise. Each of these activities is part of managing the body God has given you. Paul tells us the body is the temple of the Holy Spirit (1 **Corinthians 6:19-20**). While he explains this as a reason to avoid sexual immorality, it is also a reason to be a good steward of the body you have been given.

During pregnancy, your body serves not only yourself, but also the child God has entrusted to your care. All the decisions that can affect your health can also affect the health of your baby. It is important to evaluate the choices we make in our lives to ensure we are being good stewards of the things God has put into our control.

God does not only want your physical body. Jeremiah understood that God directed the very steps of his life (**Jeremiah 10:23**). We see this idea repeated in the New Testament. Our lives should be lived for God, not for ourselves (**2 Corinthians 5:15**). God even goes one step further. He does not merely own people, but the whole world and everything in it belongs to him (**Psalm 24:1**). Stewardship then becomes an issue to be considered for our health, the path we take and the world around us.

Being a steward is not always easy. The wicked servant in the parable of the talents feared his master's wrath if he made a poor choice. It can be even more difficult when you see no immediate results for your work. It can be a struggle to continually choose to do the right thing (**Galatians 6:9**). It is easy to tell ourselves the little things like what you eat for lunch do not matter. But Jesus understood that if we are not faithful with the small things, we will not be faithful with the big things (**Luke 16:10-12**).

Discussion Questions:

How would thinking of your body as belonging to God change the decisions you make every day?

What does the way you manage the things God has given you say about you

Do your goals line up with God's goals for you?

Add your personal insights

Unit One
Stewardship
My Thoughts...

Productive or Unproductive

A healthy concern can be productive, encouraging you to make the healthiest decisions for yourself and your baby. Such concern is a motivator, moving us to do the things God desires for us to do.

Learning how to handle the challenges of labor is what drives most women to childbirth classes. Labor and birth have become so separate from our lives that very few women have actually seen a birth before their first child is born. Because of this, a normal healthy concern to be as prepared as possible can be helpful.

Yet for some women, concern becomes an unproductive fear, paralyzing them from making decisions or enjoying the blessings of a pregnancy. In addition to preventing proper preparation, such fears can cause problems during a labor. The female body is designed to stop labor in unsafe situations. Regardless of the cause, fear is a trigger for stopping labor.

There are a lot of unknowns in labor because you are not in control. Yet you can take comfort in knowing God is in control. Even if the task set before you is difficult, God will give you the strength to come through it.

Do not confuse a lack of concern with trusting God. Judge how much you are trusting God by looking at every area of your life, not just pregnancy. It is possible to feel a lack of concern because you are choosing to avoid the reality of the situation. Avoidance may be another form of fear.

In short, your faith in God is not exhibited by the lack of concern for labor, but in your continuing to act according to the will of God regardless of what is going on around you.

More Than Meets the Eye

You are more than just a bag of flesh. You are a body and spirit, and both parts of you will be challenged during labor. You will learn to master physical comfort techniques with a little practice. It will take much more than practice to master spiritual comfort.

Spiritual comfort comes from peace and trust, perseverance and resting in the Lord. These are more than simple attitudes to adopt during labor; they are the evidence of a heart that loves and serves God alone.

Your spiritual comfort must be built before labor begins. It comes from spending time with God through Bible reading and prayer. It comes from confessing any sins you may have hidden in your heart, being honest about fears and thanking God for who he is and what he has done. Spiritual comfort comes from recognizing the true power and nature of God, and finding rest in him alone.

Spiritual comfort will not come from doing the "right things" in labor; it only exists where the heart is truly serving God.

24

Title: **Scripture Insight**

Page: 25

Type: Discussion

Purpose: Explore scriptural concepts for pregnancy and birth

Time: 15 minutes or as homework

Discussion: What a revolutionary concept to consider. Menstruation and sex existed in the Garden of Eden. While life was perfect; before sin entered the world; while everyone was still holy, the cycles of a woman's fertility existed. Neither dirty nor sinful; not a punishment, but instead a way to fulfill the plan of God. A way for Eve to participate in the miracle of life.

God did not curse the man and the woman. God did not even remove from them the responsibilities he gave them. He allowed the man to continue to work the fields and he allowed the woman to continue to give birth. However, the work involved in both tasks would be increased. The work may be difficult, but neither would be impossible to complete.

What a different picture this is from what is often attributed to Eve. After giving birth Eve did not see the process as a curse. She was amazed by the miracle she had just experienced. She understood God had allowed her to continue to be a part of bringing new life into the world.

Facilitating: It may be helpful to have Bible study tools available when discussing this material. Allow skeptics to look up the passages and the original words used for themselves. Let them see the word that is often translated as pain for Eve was translated as work for Adam. Let them explore the rest of the Bible to learn how this word is translated in other instances.

Having misunderstood scripture means only that you did not have all the information. Similarly, it is difficult to read the Bible without placing the values of your society into the text.

Questions: What are some reasons this text may have evolved into a belief that childbirth was a curse on all women?

What happens when you think and believe childbirth is a curse?

What effect does reading this these verses have on your understanding of fertility?

Workbook Page 25

Scripture Insight

Read Genesis 2-4, answering these questions.

1. When did God create human reproduction?

2. When then, were menstruation, pregnancy and child birth designed?

3. What or who did God curse?

4. What were the consequences for the man?

5. What were the consequences for the woman?

6. Compare the general impressions of the work of gardening to the work of giving birth.

7. What was Eve's response to the birth of a child?

To Pray About

How has your life demonstrated good stewardship, either during this pregnancy or before?

What unique opportunities for stewardship have arisen during this pregnancy?

What areas are the most difficult for you to practice good stewardship?

Unit One
Stewardship
My Thoughts...
Peace and Strength

Psalm 119:165

Isaiah 30:15

John 14:27

Philippians 4:6-7

Philippians 4:13

2 Timothy 1:7

25

Overview

Labor is not something that happens to a woman. Giving birth is an active process, and the woman giving birth has the ability to work with her body or to hinder her body. Understanding the ways to work with her body can help her to stay as comfortable as possible and to give birth normally.

There is a wide variety of techniques available for a woman to use during labor. Families must understand when each technique may be helpful and how to be prepared to make good decisions during the actual labor. This unit will give them the background information about labor and comfort measures to help them be prepared.

Keep this class focused on trying a wide variety of comfort measures rather than becoming an expert in any techniques. The families will need to determine which types of comfort measures work the best for them, and can then focus efforts on those techniques. However, remind the families that even comfort measures that seem ineffective now may be helpful in labor.

Help families discover the difference between comfort and peace. Families may be uncomfortable during labor, but they can still have peace as they labor. Families may also labor comfortably but have no peace about the process.

Unit Goals

After this class your students should be able to:
• Describe the process of labor
• Demonstrate techniques to stay comfortable in labor
• Explain ways to use their faith during labor

Suggested Reading

Christian Childbirth Handbook

God's Design for Childbirth
Childbirth Pain
Staying Comfortable

Lord of Birth

Why is Labor so Bad?
Inviting God to Your Baby's Birth

Birthing Naturally Web site

Comfort Techniques
Labor Progress

Sample Schedule

Time	Activity	Page
15 Minutes	No Rules, No Limits	28
30 Minutes	The Process of Labor	29-31
55 Minutes	Staying Comfortable	32-34
15 Minutes	Emotional Comfort	35-36

Overview

This unit focuses on learning how to manage labor in comfort and peace. The process of labor and what you can do to stay as comfortable as possible during labor are important things to understand. To effectively use any of these comfort measures in labor, you will need to practice them enough that you can do them while in pain and in a distracting environment.

Spiritual comfort does not come from practicing tricks and techniques to use when life is not going your way. Peace cannot be practiced or taught. True peace comes from a heart in a right relationship with God. For this reason your spiritual preparation for labor can and does influence your comfort during labor.

Discussion Points

✓ Understanding the normal process of labor can help you determine what types of physical comfort measures to use at different times in labor.

✓ Taking the time to discover the uniqueness of your body can help you understand what comfort measures will be most effective for you during labor.

✓ It may be possible that maintaining a quiet and undisturbed atmosphere could help you labor. It may also be possible that maintaining the right attitude can help you labor.

✓ Do not misinterpret the source of the power. The environment does not determine the spirit; it is the Spirit that determines the environment. You can have peace in the midst of a storm.

✓ Deep abdominal breathing (the breath of life) provides your body with the oxygen it needs to labor while it also works to keep your spirit at peace.

Self-Study

✎ Make a list of your most painful experiences. For each experience, write out the types of comfort measures you tried and how well they worked. What does this teach you about your body, and your needs for comfort?

✎ Do a topical study on God as your comforter. In what ways does God provide comfort for his people?

✎ Ask friends and family about the comfort measures they used in labor. How did they prepare to use them? How effective were they? What can you learn from their experiences?

Scripture Checklist

- ❏ Isaiah 30:15
- ❏ Psalm 119:165
- ❏ John 14:27
- ❏ Philippians 4:6-8
- ❏ Isaiah 26:3
- ❏ 2 Timothy 1:7
- ❏ Philippians 4:13
- ❏ Ecclesiastes 3:1-8
- ❏
- ❏
- ❏
- ❏

Suggested Readings

Lord of Birth

Why is Labor so Bad?
Inviting God to Your Baby's Birth

Christian Childbirth Handbook

God's Design for Childbirth
Childbirth Pain
Staying Comfortable

Birthing Naturally Web site

Comfort Techniques
Labor Progress

27

Title: **No Rules, No Limits**

Page: 28

Type: Reflection

Purpose: Identify the unique things each family needs to feel relaxed, comfortable and confident during labor.

Time: Up to 15 minutes

Directions: Explain to the families that each individual is unique and needs different conditions to feel relaxed, comfortable and confident. Ask them to share a time when they felt comfortable and confident. What was it that helped them feel comfort in that situation?

Inform the families they will have a few minutes to think about their ideal birth. They should think about where they will be, who will be with them, what they will do, what they will feel like, what they wear, what they hear…try to incorporate all 5 senses. After a short reflection time, ask families to write, draw or otherwise record their ideal birth.

After families have written their ideal births, have them share a few highlights. This allows them to see the differences in what each family needs to feel comfortable. You might start the conversation by saying, "I would love to hear some ideal births. Would anyone be willing to share?"

Facilitating: Take the time to share ideal births. Understanding that each family is unique in what it needs is the first step to forming a usable birth plan. Once families realize they cannot assume the hospital staff, doctors, nurses and midwives know what they need, they can begin to comprehend the importance of writing a birth plan.

Give your families the freedom to express their ideal birth in the way that is most comfortable to them. Some may draw a picture, some may write bullet points and others may write several paragraphs. The idea is not to have any particular finished product, but for the family to begin to understand themselves.

If time is short, this activity can be assigned as homework.

Materials: Creative writing materials (colored pencils, markers, stickers)

Scripture: Isaiah 26:3
You will keep in perfect peace him whose mind is steadfast, because he trusts in you.

It is important to remember that peace comes from God, not from the circumstances. You can have a wonderful birth, even if it is not ideal.

Unit Two
Labor Comfort

My Thoughts...

No Rules, No Limits

Use this space to write, draw, outline or otherwise record your ideal birth.
There are no restrictions on where you are, who is with you or what you can do.
Simply think about what, in your mind, would be the perfect way for your baby
to be born into your family.

28

Title:	**Normal Labor**
Page:	29
Type:	Lecture
Purpose:	List indicators of progress during labor.
Time:	10 minutes
Directions:	This page is for note taking while you explain the averages for the indicators of progress in labor.

For each measure, explain what it is, how the measuring happens and what averages are for each stage of labor.

Use the times under the contraction heading to have the families practice timing contractions. If families have understood how to time a contraction, they should be able to predict the next two contractions. Ask families to complete that part on their own, sharing answers as a group. |
| Facilitating: | Be sure families understand there are no hard and fast rules about how fast labor happens or how long you are at each stage. Even these measures can only use averages to get a picture of how labor is progressing.

If you are familiar with the emotional signposts of labor, understand there will be a time to discuss that later. At this point simply be sure the families understand the measures which are likely to be used.

You can have families copy the averages for each stage of labor under each stage on the next page. |
| Materials: | Labor charts or diagrams
Model uterus, pelvis, baby |
| Scripture: | Ecclesiastes 3:1
There is a time for everything, and a season for every activity under heaven:

Every labor is different. Every labor progresses at its own rate. You cannot control how fast or slow your labor happens. You can try to work with your body to allow labor to happen as quickly as possible, but even with the best circumstances, your labor may always be slower than a friends.

You cannot force labor to go faster or slower than it needs to without causing problems. There is usually a reason a slow labor is slow. It is better to try to address the reason before attempting general labor speeding techniques. |

Normal Labor

What does each of the following indicators reveal about the labor process?
What are the generally accepted averages during normal labor?

Contractions

Calculate the frequency and duration of these contractions. Predict the next few contractions if the pattern continues.

Begins	Ends	Frequency	Duration
8:45:20	8:46:20		
8:47:19	8:48:20		
8:49:17	8:50:20		

Dilation

Effacement

Station

Cervical Position

Sketch a cervix at different stages of labor. How does the cervix change as labor progresses?

Unit Two
Labor Comfort
My Thoughts...

29

Title: **The Experience of Labor**

Page: 30

Type: Discussion

Purpose: List mother's needs and ways to stay comfortable at each stage of labor.

Time: 10 minutes

Directions: This page is for note taking while you talk about the stages of labor. You have already discussed the indicators of progress; now you will describe the stages in terms of physical and emotional indicators

Begin with pre-labor. Ask families to share ideas about what the mother feels physically and emotionally. Work through each stage of labor this way up to transition. Describe the variation in lengths.

Facilitating: An alternative presentation method is to use a birth video or read a birth story. Ask the families to describe what the mother did at each stage of labor. Ask them to list ways her behavior and needs changed.

An alternative presentation method for families already familiar with comfort measures is to pass out cards with comfort measures on them to small groups of students. Ask families to group the comfort measures according to which stage of labor they feel they would be most helpful. Have groups share their answers, and why they selected specific techniques for specific stations with the whole class.

There is no one hardest part of labor. Every woman experiences labor based on her body, her baby's position and the speed of her labor. What was difficult for one woman may not be difficult for another.

Average is not the same as normal. Think, for example, of the average height for women. How wide is the range of "normal" from average? Do short women need to be raised with special shoes to make them normal? Do tall women need to slouch to be normal? Average and normal are two related, but completely different terms.

Materials: Birth video or story cards
Comfort Measure Cards

Scripture: 2 Corinthians 12:9-10
But he said to me, "My grace is sufficient for you, for my power is made perfect in weakness." Therefore I will boast all the more gladly about my weaknesses, so that Christ's power may rest on me. That is why, for Christ's sake, I delight in weaknesses, in insults, in hardships, in persecutions, in difficulties. For when I am weak, then I am strong.

Remember it is not your strength, but God's.

Unit Two
Labor Comfort
My Thoughts...

The Experience of Labor

Each stage of labor has specific physical and emotional characteristics that define it. By understanding how to interpret the signs of progress, you will be better able to make decisions about how to handle your labor. Also, each stage of labor has different challenges. Knowing ways to manage your comfort level can help you give birth with the least intervention possible.

Identify the characteristics and challenges of each stage of labor.

Pre-Labor

Early First Stage

Late First Stage

Transition

30

Title:	**The Labor Clock**
Page:	31
Type:	Worksheet
Purpose:	Explain the timing of the average labor.
Time:	10 minutes
Directions:	The circle is to be the outline of a clock. Use lines to distinguish the length of time at each stage of labor. The line at 12:00 is to be the start and end of the "average" 12 hour labor.
	Have your families count backwards from the end of labor. How long would be a normal, but not necessarily ideal, amount of time to push? Because average varies, families should pick a time within the range of normal; this may be thirty minutes or three hours. Families should put a line at the time that will represent the start of the pushing time they have selected. For example, if they selected one hour, a line is drawn at eleven o'clock. Have families do the same for transition and active labor. The rest of the time is early labor. Have families share their clock so other families can see what normal labors may look like.
	After filling in the times, have your families write the name in each stage. You should have already talked about what a woman may feel at each stage. Using that knowledge, fill in mother's needs for each stage. Share ideas with the group.
Facilitating:	An alternative activity is to represent labor as a time line. Families can select the time for each stage of labor themselves, or draw them at random from a set of choices you have prepared.
	In a group class, it is expected to have different amounts of time for the stages of labor, but the amounts of time should be realistic.
	If time allows, create one clock as a whole group. Then have individual families create their own clocks.
Materials:	"Average" lengths of labor stages chart
Scripture:	Philippians 4:13
I can do everything through him who gives me strength.
	The secret to being content is not getting what you want, but understanding that even when what you get is not ideal, God gives you strength to get through it.

The Labor Clock

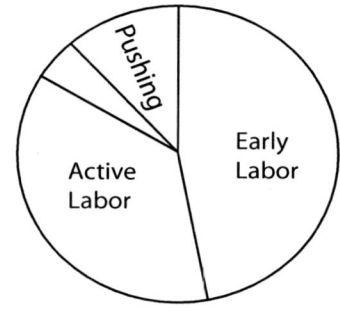

If the average labor is 12 hours, you can graphically represent an average labor on a standard clock face. In this exercise you will graph one normal labor. There is no right or wrong here. Normal lengths of labor stages are highly variable.

Using the circle, the line at 12:00 will be the point the baby is born. Now count backwards. What is an average pushing time? Draw a line from the center to the point on the clock that makes that time (see example). How long is an average transition? How long might a normal active labor be?

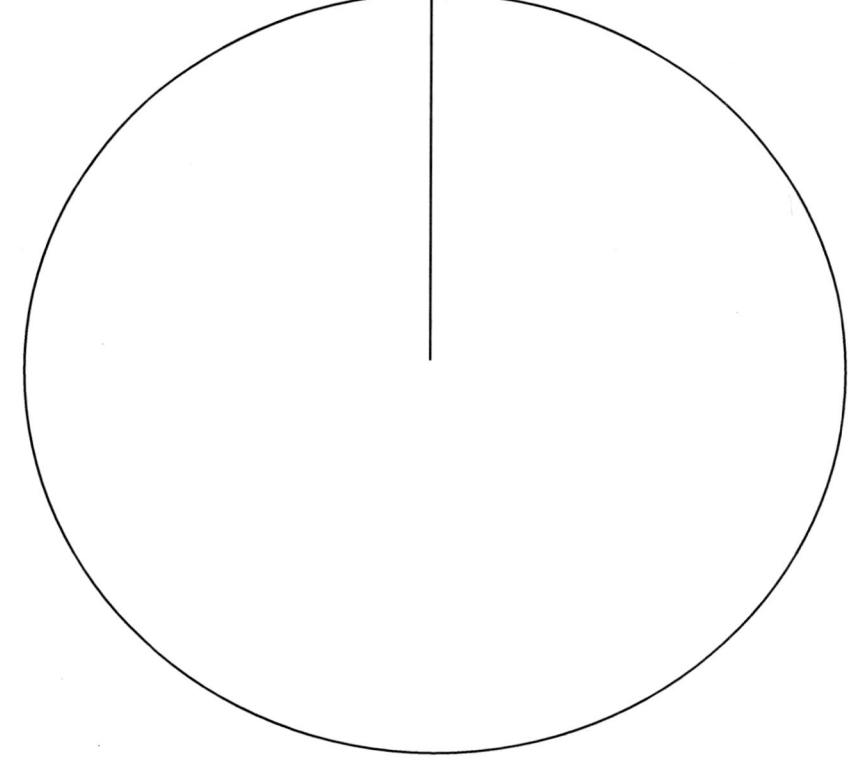

Discussion Question:
What might help you stay comfortable during each stage of labor?

31

Title:	**Positions for Labor**
Page:	32
Type:	Guided Discovery
Purpose:	List positions for labor and their benefits.
Time:	15 minutes
Directions:	Positions are listed on the worksheet, grouped according to type of position. Have students read through the list quickly before attempting any position.
	Show the position to the families, asking them to perform the position as well. As they assume each position, ask them what could be done while in this position to help them remain comfortable. Could the mother sip water, rock her hips or use a heating pad? What parts of the mother could be massaged?
	Try as many positions as possible. Encourage families to write notes about what they like or do not like about positions after trying them.
Facilitating:	Have equipment ready for families to try, such as a birth ball, a chair, a stool. You may also want to give them access to stairs or a bathroom.
	An alternate presentation would be to set up stations around the room with directions for different positions to try. Allow the families to move about the room as they desire or run a rotation schedule. Be available to answer questions.
	Encourage families to think about their homes this week. What positions can they use, and what places in their home will work well for different positions?
	You may find it easier to talk about positions and physical comfort measures at the same time.
Materials:	Birth Ball Chairs Floor mats Labor Position Station Cards

Unit Two
Labor Comfort
My Thoughts...

Positions for Labor

Try each of these positions. Record your thoughts on page 37.

Upright Positions allow gravity to increase the intensity of the contractions naturally, while minimizing the discomfort.

Standing

Walking

Leaning against a wall

Dangling in someone's arms

Slow dancing

Leaning over a chair

Kneeling Positions take pressure off your pelvic floor and allow the baby to change positions.

Over a chair

Over a birth ball

Into someone's lap

Over the side of a tub

Over the side of the bed

Over the end of the bed

Sitting Positions allow your body to work with gravity while allowing you to rest.

Chair, forward or backward

Beanbag Chair

Birth Ball

Floor, tailor style

Toilet

Rocking chair

Positions that give you the freedom to move your pelvis may help your baby to rotate, allowing for a faster labor.

• Try pelvic rocking in any of the upright or kneeling positions.
• Try slow dancing with a partner for support
• Sway your hips back and forth during contractions
• Try lunging forward with your foot on a chair or stool
• Try walking in between or during contractions
• Rock your hips in a figure eight during contractions
• Rock your torso back and forth as you sit

32

Title:	**Physical Comfort Measures for Labor**
Page:	33
Type:	Problem Solving
Purpose:	Understand when and how to use a variety of comfort measures.
Time:	20 minutes
Directions:	Begin by asking families to make a list of all the ways they have managed pain on a white board. Ask them to think of the pain of a headache, being hungry or tired, consitpation, burns, broken bones or any other pain they have experienced.
	After creating the list, introduce the page to families. Explain that everything on their list can be tried during labor; discuss any comfort measures from the page not included in the list they made. Demonstrate comfort measures where appropriate.
	Return to the Labor Clock used earlier in the class. Using the information on positions and comfort measures, have families list things they can do in each stage of labor to remain comfortable.
	After they have listed their selections, have them share their ideas with the group making suggestions for more effective uses if necessary.
Facilitating:	It is important to remind families that they are already experts on the pain they feel and what they need to manage their pain. During labor they may be under stress, which makes it difficult to remember some of the things they can do, so keeping a list can be helpful.
	The list in the workbook is not intended to be an exhaustive listing of comfort measures, but rather a listing of major categories of comfort techniques. If time allows, have families list additional comfort measures and variations of each category.
Materials:	Hot or cold packs
Massage tools
Water bottles
Scripture:	John 14:27
Peace I leave with you; my peace I give you. I do not give to you as the world gives. Do not let your hearts be troubled and do not be afraid.
	Comfort and peace are not the same. Even if nothing you do is working to keep you comfortable, God can still give you peace.

My Thoughts...

Physical Comfort Measures for Labor

There are many types of pain and discomfort women may feel during labor. For those not wishing to use pain relieving medications, or those waiting for the medication to take effect, the following methods of pain relief may be useful.

Try each of these comfort measures. Record your thoughts on page 37.

Heat / Cold can be applied to the area experiencing pain. The result is a dulling sensation of the pain.

Massage techniques can be used to relieve a sore back or any aching muscle.

Showers can be used to help you relax. If the stream of water is placed over the uncomfortable part of the body, the pain may lessen.

Baths can alleviate discomforts on many parts of the body at one time by relieving the weight of your body, providing heat to the areas experiencing discomfort and promoting relaxation.

Patterned Breathing can distract you from the discomfort you feel, and bring your attention away from the contraction.

Vocalization in the form of moaning, sighing, counting, singing, chanting or praying may help you relax while distracting you from your contractions. Many women find matching the volume of the vocalization to the intensity of the contraction helps them remain in control.

Abdominal Breathing helps promote relaxation and provides the body with more oxygen than chest breathing. This helps prevent fatigue and allows the muscles to work at their best.

Sleep between contractions or during early labor helps increase your stamina. You will not sleep through the birth, so sleep if you are able.

Using the Bathroom can relieve pelvic pressure by keeping the bowel and bladder empty. As the cervix dilates, you may not be able to discern if the pressure is from the cervix or a full bladder. Keeping the bladder empty can prevent some pain.

Drinking and Eating prevent dehydration and fatigue, both of which can make the contractions seem more intense and painful.

33

Title:	**Abdominal Breathing**
Page:	34
Type:	Guided Discovery
Purpose:	Correctly perform abdominal breathing.
Time:	5-10 minutes
Directions:	Have families sit on the floor with the mother's abdomen visible and within reach of her partner, perhaps lying on her side or reclining on her partner.
	Ask mothers to take five big breaths while the partner watches the mother's chest and abdomen. What part of her body moves and how does it move?
	Explain how to breath abdominally, and why it is the preferred method for labor.
	Ask mothers to take five big breaths again, this time with the mother and partner placing a hand on mother's abdomen. They should feel her abdomen gently rising and falling. Ask families to share how this is different.
	Once mothers are comfortable, ask them to meditate on one of the verses listed on the worksheet while they breathe abdominally for 2 minutes.
Facilitating:	This is an easy exercise to encourage families to begin touching each other, and may work best in the first class if you have time for it.
	Breathing should be slow and deep, but not so slow and deep mothers become light-headed. Be sure they change positions slowly after this exercise.
Materials:	Labor scripture cards
Scripture:	Job 12:10 In his hand is the life of every creature and the breath of all mankind.
	Job 33:4 The Spirit of God has made me; the breath of the Almighty gives me life.
	John 20:21-22 Again Jesus said, "Peace be with you! As the Father has sent me, I am sending you." And with that he breathed on them and said, "Receive the Holy Spirit.

Unit Two
Labor Comfort
My Thoughts...

Abdominal Breathing

Not only does abdominal breathing enhance relaxation, it also increases the lung capacity. This means there is more oxygen for you and your baby. Abdominal breathing also uses less of your energy.

To learn to breathe abdominally, do this:

Breathe in deeply, if your shoulders rise, you are chest breathing not abdominal breathing.

Breathe in deeply again, this time try to push your abdominal muscles out as you breathe in.

As you exhale, your abdominal muscles should pull back in.

How does abdominal breathing feel different from the way you normally breathe?

Spend a few minutes meditating on these scripture verses.
How does God use them to speak to you?

Job 12:10

Job 33:4

John 20:21-22

When to use Abdominal Breathing

You should use abdominal breathing throughout most of your labor. However, you may find it most useful when you:

• Feel "out of control"
• Have become frightened or stressed
• Are having difficulties relaxing
• Have lost your "focus"

34

Title: **Spiritual Comfort Measures for Labor**

Page: 35

Type: Discussion

Purpose: Master skills for emotional comfort during labor.

Time: 15 minutes

Directions: Begin by asking families what they expect emotionally during labor. Spend some time talking about why they expect to feel that way.

                If no one brings it up, ask the families what they normally do to manage emotional stresses such as fear, anxiety or embarrassment. Lead the discussion to Christian disciplines listed on the sheet.

                Remind families that these disciplines should be practiced regularly, not just during times of stress. A peaceful spirit comes from being in a right relationship with God. This does not mean you will not experience fear or anxiety, but that you will have the strength of God to handle it.

Facilitating: Though all the spiritual disciplines are helpful, families will find they are each unique in the way they connect with God best. If a woman feels closest to God while reading scripture, she may find that to be most helpful during labor.

                Using spiritual disciplines during labor may look different than when not in labor because of the amount of work labor requires. Encourage families to begin experimenting with techniques such as repeating short prayers written on index cards or using one of the other suggestions. Not only will this be helpful during labor, but it will give families ways to stay connected with God during the busy first weeks of a new baby in the home.

Materials: Labor meditation cards
                Scripture list or cards

Scripture: Isaiah 30:15
                This is what the Sovereign LORD, the Holy One of Israel, says: "In repentance and rest is your salvation,
                in quietness and trust is your strength,
                but you would have none of it.

                It is human nature to try to make our lives as comfortable as possible. The reality of life is that we seldom wait for God to provide his comfort. Instead we fight for what we want, struggle to make sure everything is perfect.

My Thoughts...

Spiritual Comfort Measures for Labor

Comfort in labor is affected by where your mind and your spirit are focused. If you are fearful, anxious or lacking trust in God, your labor may be hindered. Unlike the physical comfort measures, spiritual comfort measures cannot be "mastered" and used during labor. Peace, confidence and faith take time to build, but once established will benefit you in every part of your life.

When you are in labor, there are ways to draw on your faith and peace of God to help you stay relaxed and confident. Just as you have a unique physical makeup, you also have a unique spiritual makeup. Some of these activities will comfort you more than others, so be sure to spend time trying each activity to see which ones help you the most. Read Isaiah 30:15, then try each of these activities. Record your thoughts on page 37.

Prayer is always good for the soul, and in labor it can be good for the body as well. Praying out loud can be used as a vocalization to match the intensity of contractions. Listening to others praying for you can give you a focus point. Pray using one of the many names used for God in the Bible; your comforter, your strength, your deliverer.

Scripture Reading gives us the chance to hear the words of God. These words can bring strength, comfort and peace. Scripture can be used as a focal point if someone else reads to you or if you read favorite verses from index cards. Reciting the verses aloud can be used as a form of vocalization, or as a distraction technique if you repeat a verse someone else reads.

Meditation can help prevent distraction, allowing you to achieve a deeper relaxation. Meditation can also be done as a form of prayer during labor. God calls us to meditate on his word, and in labor you might find it helpful to meditate on the miracle happening in your body.

Praise and Worship can help you stay focused on God. Music helps to establish a mood and is allowed at most birthing places.

Confession helps to keep us in a right relationship with God. Our sins have a disastrous effect on our relationship with God. Usually, we begin to feel guilt as a consequence of our sin. This guilt encourages us to return to the Lord. But when left unconfessed, that guilt can cause us to "hide" from God just like Adam and Eve in the garden.

35

Title: **Love Languages in Labor**

Page: 36

Type: Discussion

Purpose: Determine personal needs for emotional comfort during labor.

Time: No more than 10 minutes

Directions: Ask if families are familiar with the concept of love languages. If not, explain or ask a family to explain.

              If anyone does not know their love language, have them read through the list on the worksheet to determine what their love language may be. This can be assigned as homework if time is tight.

              Ask families to offer suggestions for comfort measures to use in labor that specifically meet their love language needs, such as massage for touch or vocalization for words of affirmation.

Facilitating: Alternative presentation would be to pass out comfort measure cards. Ask small groups or families to place comfort measure cards into groups according to their love language.

              Not every comfort measure is going to work for every family. The point here is to help families identify the types of comfort measures that are likely to be the most helpful during labor. Giving birth is not a psychosis, and the woman in labor does not suddenly become someone different. Instead, she will become more of the person she was created to be because she will be too tired and focused to behave in ways society teaches us to behave.

              Families should not limit their practice to the comfort measures most likely to help because additional factors such as the position of the baby and speed of labor can affect what the mother needs to stay comfortable and confident. Having a wide variety of tools available can help families overcome challenges during labor.

Materials: Comfort measure cards
              Love Languages Book

My Thoughts...

Love Languages in Labor

Few women go into labor realizing the strongest comfort measure is the love and encouragement of those supporting her.

Dr. Gary Chapman has given us a tool to understand each other with his Five Love Languages. Dr. Chapman suggests everyone has a way in which they give and receive love most powerfully. He calls it their love language. Knowing your spouse's love language allows you to focus your efforts at showing love into those areas, which communicate love to him or her most effectively. This principle holds true even through the rigors of labor.

Which of these love languages sounds most like yours?

Quality Time:
Some women feel loved when their companions choose to be with them rather than participating in another activity. For this woman, the simple act of shutting off the television so you can talk with her speaks volumes about how valuable she is to you. To love this woman in labor, you must prevent yourself from becoming distracted and preoccupied by work, telephones, hospital procedures or other concerns.

Words of Affirmation:
Every woman needs to be told how great she is doing, but for a woman whose love language is words of affirmation, your silence during labor tells her she is alone. To love this woman in labor, you must remind her after every contraction how much you love her, how strong she is, how great she is handling labor, or how much you appreciate what she is doing.

Gifts:
For some women, the fact that someone took the time to make or purchase something for them fills their heart with joy. Although you cannot run out to purchase gifts during the labor, you can prepare ahead of time. Putting together a small photo album, a collection of poems, or a CD with favorite songs, lets this woman feel how important her laboring is to you.

Acts of Service:
When a laboring woman has the acts of service love language, everything you do to help her shows how much you care. To love her in labor, you cannot allow yourself to sit at her side while the nurses do everything. You must offer her sips of water or ice, retrieve cool or warm cloths for her face, neck and back, and be her shoulder to lean on when contractions overwhelm her.

Physical Touch:
Although most women find massage of some sort comforting in labor, some women need to be touched. For these women a back rub is an expression of your love and devotion. If she gets to the point that touching her body is no longer comfortable, you can just hold her hand.

In labor, a variety of comfort measures and pain coping techniques may need to be tried. Understanding your love language allows those with you in labor to focus their efforts on the techniques that not only keep you comfortable, but also demonstrate their love to you.

Discussion:
Can you predict helpful comfort measures based on your love language?

36

Title:	**Comfort Measures Assessment**
Page:	37
Type:	Reflection
Purpose:	Identify personal needs for relaxation.
Time:	Homework
Directions:	Present the worksheet to families. Ask them to rate each of the comfort measures tried during class. Explain that it helps them to assess where they need the most practice, and what techniques are most helpful to them.
	Encourage them to continue to fill this form out before the next class
Facilitating:	It will take time for families to complete this worksheet, and not all comfort measures on the sheet will have been presented in this class. Encourage them to complete this assessment over the next few weeks.

My Thoughts...

Comfort Measures Assessment

You have been working on learning a wide variety of comfort measures for labor. Because every woman is different, your response to the various techniques will be unique. Completing this assessment will help you determine which strategies are most likely to be beneficial during labor.

	Comfort and confidence in my ability to do this			Success at managing pain and discomfort		
Technique	**Low**	**Med**	**High**	**Low**	**Med**	**High**
Abdominal Breathing						
Progressive Relaxation						
Massage						
Meditation						
Visualization						
Vocalization						
Standing or Walking						
Slow Dancing						
Leaning Forward						
Sitting on Birth Ball						
Reading						
Dangling						
Effleurage						
Hip Squeeze						
Reclining or lying						
Kneeling or hands-knees						
Patterned breathing						
Counter pressure						
Hot or cold packs						
Warm shower						
Warm bath						
Talking with someone						
Distraction						
Receiving encouragement						
Physical Touch						
Music						
Prayer						
Scripture Reading						
Meditation						
Praise / Worship						

37

Workbook Page 38 contains two devotional thoughts families can read.

Notes on **Scripture Checklist** from page 27

Many families mistakenly aim for physical comfort during labor when what they really want is peace. There is a tremendous difference between the peace God gives, and the peace we can achieve on our own. Often, we grasp for peace in ways that are opposite of the ways God intends to give us peace (**Isaiah 20:15-16**). Peace from God comes in many ways we do not understand (**Psalm 119:165**). The world expects peace from perfect circumstances. Jesus, Paul and Isaiah all remind us that peace comes from God, not from the things happening around us (**John 14:27; Philippians 4:6-8; Isaiah 26:3**).

While we are not able to build our own peace, we are also not called to sit helplessly. Paul explains that God has given us a spirit of power, love and self-discipline (**2 Timothy 1:7**). It is OK to try to improve the situation. Just be careful not to fall into the trap of believing that changing the situation will instantly give you peace. In fact, God can give you peace even if all your attempts to change the situation are unproductive. By the power of God, Paul learned to be content in any circumstance (**Philippians 4:13**)

Discussion Questions:

What is the difference between peace and comfort?

Does God promise comfort?

Is it possible to be comfortable, but not have peace?

Add your personal insights

Unit Two
Labor Comfort
My Thoughts...

A Deeper Knowing

Understanding the normal process of labor can help you determine what types of comfort measures are effective at different times during labor. There are some techniques useful for speeding labor, others useful for a backache in labor and still others that can be helpful when you feel tense.

Knowing the variety of comfort measures is only the first step. Taking the time to discover the uniqueness of your body can help you understand what comfort measures are most useful for you.

Both showers and baths can have beneficial effects in labor. They can both help ease a sore back, encourage relaxation and make you more comfortable. Yet, you probably enjoy one better than the other—and knowing which you prefer is part of the key to a deeper understanding of comfort measures.

If you are a woman who finds comfort in talking about what is happening, you may choose to talk longer into your labor than most other women.

If you are a woman who prefers silence, you may choose not to use music during labor.

If you are a woman who tenses when her feet are touched, you may want to identify other parts of your body to be massaged during labor.

If you are a woman who is constantly moving, positions that limit your mobility may be less helpful for you during labor.

It all comes down to knowing who you are. Do not expect something to work for you because it worked for someone else. God created you uniquely, and it is only you who knows what really works to help you feel comfortable.

Once you have explored the different comfort measures, you will be able to share with your labor partners what are the most effective techniques for you.

God as Comforter

We have a wonderful model of a comforter in God. As early as the story of Adam (Genesis 2:20-22), we see a God who is concerned about meeting the needs of his people. God responds to Adam's lack of a companion by making Eve.

Further into the book of Genesis, we see God comforting a forlorn Haggar by meeting both her physical needs and her emotional needs (Genesis 21:17-19). He provides water for her to drink and reassurance that Ishmael will become a strong nation.

God sends comfort to Elijah by providing food and rest. After Elijah's physical needs have been met, God meets his emotional needs by reassuring him he is not alone (1 Kings 19).

It is wonderful to know God cares about our comfort. It is important to remember God seeks to meet our physical and emotional needs. As you practice comfort measures, be sure to learn techniques to bring physical and emotional comfort. Do not underestimate the importance of the emotional comfort you feel knowing God is your strength even during labor.

38

Title: **Scripture Insight**

Page: 39

Type: Discussion

Purpose: Explore scriptural concepts for pregnancy and birth

Time: 15 minutes or as homework

Discussion: Understanding progress in labor requires understanding how the entire body works. Labor is not simply a cervix opening. Labor uses every part of a woman's body.

Her endocrine system is regulating levels of hormones to increase the strength of her contractions.

Her circulatory system is moving these hormones throughout her body.

Her skeletal system is stretching and expanding to make room for the baby through the pelvis.

Her muscles are supporting her body and preventing the downward force of contractions from pushing her entire abdominal contents through her pelvis.

Her nervous system recognizes the changes in pressure and signals her muscles to move to help accommodate the baby's position.

Her digestive system empties her bowel to allow as much room as possible for the baby.

Her respiratory system responds to the increased work by increasing the rate and depth of her breathing, ensuring she and her baby are well oxygenated.

Questions: If labor uses every part of a woman's body, why might the cervical dilation be the only measure used to estimate progress?

How might adding an outside force to open the cervix affect the labor process?

In what ways does the baby cooperate with the work of the mother during labor?

Workbook Page 39

Scripture Insight

Read Romans 12:3-8.

1. What does it mean to be holistic?

2. What is the value of a holistic view of the body of Christ?

3. What is the value of a holistic view of the human body?

4. Explain the dangers of understanding labor as solely a work of the uterus.

5. How do other parts of the body cooperate to accomplish birth?

6. Describe the ways a labor support team works together as a body.

To Pray About

What do you need to feel comfort?

What prevents you from feeling comfortable?

How has God been your comforter?

What areas are you in need of comfort today?

My Thoughts...

Strength and Confidence

Psalm 51:10-12

Psalm 73:26

Psalm 119:50

Isaiah 26:3

2 Corinthians 3:4

39

87

Overview

Mother and baby are two unique individuals, but must work in harmony to accomplish the birth. As mother's body pushes against baby; baby pushes back against mother, stretching and opening first the cervix and then the vaginal canal. The process of pushing gives us two lessons for new parents.

Lesson one is accepting that your child is a unique individual. You must be willing to let go, to allow your child to be the person God made him/her to be. Mothers sometimes report they hold back in labor because they do not want to lose the connection they have with their baby.

Lesson two is that no matter what you do, you cannot force a person to be or do what you want them to do. Sometimes babies are in positions that make pushing slow or difficult. It takes patience and humility to work in a way that helps your baby change positions so you can complete the task together.

Unit Goals

After finishing the material in this unit, your students should be able to:

- Demonstrate good pushing positions.
- Explain two pushing methods.
- Describe the proper way to do Kegel exercises.

Suggested Reading

Christian Childbirth Handbook

Second Stage
Third Stage

Birthing Naturally Web site

Comfort Techniques
Labor Progress

Sample Schedule

Time	Activity	Page
30 Minutes	Second and Third Stage Labor	42-43
30 Minutes	How to Push	44-45
45 Minutes	Staying Comfortable	46-47

Overview

The process of pushing happens slowly as you work in response to your body's urges to push. During this time you must maintain a humble attitude, willing to let yourself be directed by the cues of your body. Think of it as a metaphor for following the direction of the Holy Spirit; when the Spirit says move, you move!

But just as in the rest of life, you cannot control the response your baby will have to your pushing. Your baby may come out quickly, or he may take more time as he molds and twists through the pelvis. Sometimes babies are in positions that prevent pushing from being effective. In this case, the mother will need to adjust herself to help her baby move into a better position. Once again, you will not be able to force your baby to change position, but will instead attempt to provide him an environment that allows him to change.

Here again we have a metaphor, this time for making an impact on someone else's life. Others are not always ready to change, and we must have the patience and humility to continue to love them unconditionally in the hope they will move into a position that makes them more willing to receive the truth.

Discussion Points

✓ The process of pushing happens slowly so the baby can mold to the pelvis. Your baby will move forward during a contraction and slip back a little between contractions.

✓ Certain positions your baby may assume will cause the pushing process to take longer than average.

✓ You cannot rush the process of pushing without increasing the risks to mother or baby. However, under some circumstances the risks of allowing the birth to happen at a slow pace are higher than the risks of rushing the process.

✓ Push in any position that is comfortable. Some positions may help pushing happen faster, others may help slow pushing down.

Self-Study

☙ Spend some time reading birth stories from the Bible. Look up the stories of Eve (Genesis 3), Hannah (1 Samuel 1), Elizabeth and Mary (Luke 1-2), Leah and Rachel (Genesis 29:31-30:24). What information can you find about the attitude of new mothers and those around them,

☙ Find out about the birth options in your area. Do you have hospitals, birth centers, access to homebirth? Can you hire a midwife, obstetrician or family doctor?

☙ Ask friends or family to share their feelings as they saw their baby for the first time. Did they experience joy or relief? Were they drawn to one feature such as eyes or hands? Did they spend hours taking pictures or talking to their new baby?

Unit Three
Greeting Baby

Scripture Checklist
❑ Isaiah 57:15
❑ Isaiah 66:9
❑ Psalm 51:16-17
❑ Proverbs 11:2
❑ James 3:13
❑ Matthew 23:12
❑
❑
❑
❑

Suggested Readings
Christian Childbirth Handbook
Second Stage
Third Stage
Birthing Naturally Web site
Comfort Techniques
Labor Progress

41

Title:	**What is Second Stage?**
Page:	42
Type:	Guided Discovery
Purpose:	Describe the process of giving birth.
Time:	10-15 minutes
Directions:	Begin by asking families what the baby does during pushing. After ideas are shared, refer families to the worksheet.
	Give families time to experiment with the model while you explain the Ferguson Reflex and Dr. Odent's Fetal Ejection Reflex
	Show families the model pelvis. You can explain to families how to find the pubic bone and the coccyx on their own bodies. Although they may not want to find these bones in class, encourage them to find them when at home. Ask them to feel how these bones move as they change positions, and show this movement with the model pelvis. What would make it easier for the baby to exit the pelvis.
	Describe the process of engagement and rotation. Using a model or by moving your own body show the positions the baby must move through to exit the pelvis.
	Explain crowning and the differences between crowning and the opening of the cervix.
Facilitating:	Families may be confused by the initial question, believing the baby is simply pushed out rather than being an active participant in the process. An alternative presentation would be to start with a video which shows transition and second stage. Center the discussion around what families are able to see in the video.
	The process is easier to understand when families are able to see models or if you mimic the position changes with your head.
Materials:	Model pelvis and baby Birth video
Scripture:	Isaiah 66:9 Do I bring to the moment of birth and not give delivery?" says the LORD. "Do I close up the womb when I bring to delivery?" says your God.
	God has designed a system of birth that works. Moreover, God is with you through childbirth. It is God who brings your child to delivery. It is God who opens the womb.

Unit Three
Greeting Baby
My Thoughts...

What is second Stage?

The cervix is opened and the baby drops into the birth canal. What is important to understand about each of these parts of second stage?

Ferguson Reflex

Fetal Ejection Reflex

Pelvis

Pelvic Inlet   Pelvic Outlet

Cardinal Movements

Crowning

42

Title: **How to Push**

Page: 43

Type: Guided Discovery

Purpose: List benefits and risks of pushing methods.

Time: 10-15 minutes

Directions: Explain to families a common concern among expectant mothers is that they will not know how to push.

You have already explained the reflexes involved in pushing. Ask families to list other reflexes (such as the need to go to the bathroom or removing your hand from a hot surface). Ask families to consider what it means for something to be a reflex. Have families share ideas about what may stop the birth reflexes.

Briefly explain both pushing methods, then let families experience both methods using a watch to time a pushing contraction. Stress to families that they are not actually to push at this time, but can still get a feel for the timing of breaths and the environment for each method.

After explaining each method of pushing, have families consider the differences between the two methods. How might these differences impact the process of giving birth? How might these differences affect the mother?

Facilitating: Consider having mothers or yourself role-play each pushing method to help them see the differences.

With the next birth video you show, ask families to figure out what pushing method the mother is using.

Be sure to review the importance of Kegel exercises for preparing the pelvic floor. Ending this section with Kegel exercises makes an easy transition to protecting the perineum.

Materials: Watch with second hand
                Birth Video

My Thoughts...

How to Push

For some women, the fear of knowing when or how to push is the biggest fear of labor. For other women, the images of births in movies and TV have given them a faulty understanding of what the pushing process actually entails.

Reflexive Pushing

When a mother is left alone to follow her body, pushing is reflexive. Usually performed with many short pushes lasting no longer than 6 seconds each. If the contraction is stronger, the mother naturally pushes harder.

Directed Pushing

When a mother is faced with the need to give birth quickly, she is directed to take a cleansing breath, inhale deeply and push as hard as she can to the count of 10. When she reaches 10, she takes a quick breath and pushes to the count of 10 again. This gives about three long, strong pushes during a contraction.

What are the differences between these two pushing methods?
Benefits and risks:

Length of pushing time:

Breathing and vocalization:

Role of the Partner:

What is the same regardless of the pushing method used?
Use of pelvic floor muscles:

Where push is directed:

Relaxing between pushing contractions:

Discussion Question:
Read Isaiah 66:9. The idea of pushing brings fear to the hearts of many women. Why do you think women are not aware of the amazing ability of their body to stretch?

43

Title:	**Protect the Perineum**
Page:	44
Type:	Buzz Group
Purpose:	List ways to keep perineal skin intact.
Time:	10 minutes
Directions:	Ask families for ideas of ways to keep the skin intact to help prevent both episiotomy and tearing. Explain how to choose oils and hand out directions for perineal massage if appropriate.
	Give families time to share the information they have about episiotomy and tearing. Offer the benefits and risks associated with each argument if families do not provide them all. Present research facts about both tearing and episiotomy.
Facilitating:	An alternative would be to have families research this topic before class, and share information as a group.
Materials:	Massage oil Perineal massage handouts
Scripture:	Isaiah 66:9 Do I bring to the moment of birth and not give delivery?" says the LORD. "Do I close up the womb when I bring to delivery?" says your God.
	God uses the imagery of birth to demonstrate his faithfulness. What does this say about the frequency of problems that naturally occur with childbirth?

Workbook Page 44

Unit Three
Greeting Baby
My Thoughts...

Protect the Perineum

The goal is to end labor with your skin as intact as possible, so prevention should be the focus. List ways to help keep the perineal skin intact.

Before labor begins

During labor

Do you know the arguments for natural tearing of the perineum? Do you know the arguments for episiotomy? What does the research support?

Tearing

Episiotomy

Research

44

95

Title:	**The Immediate Postpartum**
Page:	45
Type:	Lecture
Purpose:	Describe the events immediately after a baby is born.
Time:	10 Minutes
Directions:	Ask families what they expect to happen immediately after their baby is born. Discuss each item, allowing families to take notes on the page.
	Highlight the options available for each event. When appropriate, offer benefits and risks of the various options.
Facilitating:	If possible, select a birth video for the previous section that demonstrates both pushing and the immediate postpartum care.
	Photographs or a model placenta and umbilical cord can help families visualize what is happening.
	If teaching a review class, ask families what they liked about the immediate postpartum. Then ask if there was anything they would like to change for this time?
Materials:	Birth Video Birth Charts Model Placenta and Umbilical Cord

Workbook Page 45

The Immediate Post Partum

Things happen quickly once your baby is born. What is important to understand about each of these events?

Hormonal Changes

Breast feeding and Bonding

Cord Cutting

Birth of the Placenta

Repair of the Perineum

My Thoughts...

45

Title: **Staying Comfortable While Pushing**

Page: 46

Type: Brainstorm

Purpose: List comfort measures to be used during pushing.

Time: 10 minutes

Directions: This sheet is organized for families to take notes.

Explain to the families they have already learned a wide variety of comfort measures which may be useful for pushing. Ask them to begin listing ways they could help a mother stay comfortable during pushing.

As ideas surface, help families categorize and expand on the topic to identify more comfort techniques. Use the page to prompt ideas if necessary.

Facilitating: Be prepared for groups who are not talkative or do not give answers by having comfort measures written on cards before class begins. Pass out the cards to the families and have them suggest ways the comfort measure can be used during pushing.

With groups who have a good understanding of birth, begin exploring how these factors may hinder the progress of a birth.

This is a discussion that can benefit from a birth video highlighting pushing.

Materials: Birth Video
Comfort Measure Cards

Unit Three
Greeting Baby
My Thoughts...

Staying Comfortable While Pushing

What does each of these have to do with staying comfortable while pushing?

Breathing and Breath Holding

Positioning

Fighting Fatigue

Lighting

Temperature (room and body)

Companions

Crowning

46

Title:	**Second Stage Positions**
Page:	47
Type:	Guided Discovery
Purpose:	List benefits of positioning for pushing.
Time:	10-15 minutes
Directions:	Describe the guidelines for a "good" pushing position. Explain to the families that any position will work, but some will work faster or slower or more comfortably than others.
	Work through each category of pushing positions, explaining variations and having families practice the position. Describe benefits for the position and potential unintended consequences.
	After giving time to practice each position, have families share thoughts. Which positions were most comfortable? Which positions needed the most help and support for the mother?
Facilitating:	Provide lots of space and any materials needed to allow families to try the positions.
	If space or equipment prohibits, set up stations to try each type of position and have families rotate after explaining and demonstrating.
Materials:	Chairs, pillows, floor mat, towel Pushing Station Markers
Scripture:	James 1:18 He chose to give us birth through the word of truth, that we might be a kind of first fruits of all he created.
	God repeatedly uses the imagery of birth to help people understand the change that happens when you follow Christ. What does this say about God and our relationship with Christ? What does this say about giving birth?

My Thoughts...

Second Stage Positions

Almost any position that is comfortable for the mother will work for pushing. However, there are benefits to using each type of position.

List potential benefits for each position.

Squatting Positions

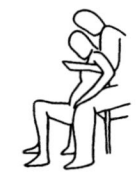

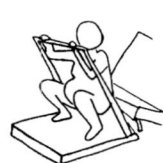

Reclining Positions

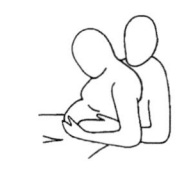

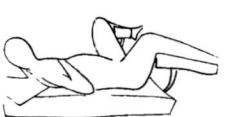

Kneeling Positions

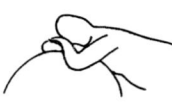

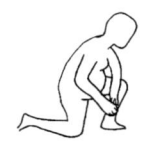

Standing Positions

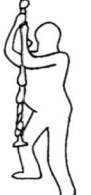

47

Workbook Page 48 contains two devotional thoughts families can read.

Notes on **Scripture Checklist** from page 41

The imagery of birth in the Bible is amazing. It is used in prophecy to help explain God's faithfulness (**Isaiah 66:9**), and the effects of fear (**Isaiah 21:3; Jeremiah 48:41; Jeremiah 30:4-6**), and even the process of change (**Matthew 24:8**). You will find a more complete listing of the places birth is used to teach in the Scripture Insight activity for Unit Six.

Just as birth was used to teach the Israelites, the process of birth can teach us. For example, the nature of second stage puts the mother in the position to follow. Even though she must do the work of pushing, she must pay attention to the cues and signals her body gives her. It will not work if she tries to push before her body says, or if she decides not to push when her body says go. This makes second stage a wonderful example of humility. The mother is strong and capable, but willingly submits to the directions of her body. She is not in control, but she is not giving up.

Humility is described as the sacrifice God expects (**Psalm 51:16-17**). God goes so far as to say he dwells with those who have contrite hearts (**Isaiah 57:15**). Humility is said to bring wisdom (**Proverbs 11:2; James 3:13**). Humility is so important to the Christian life, Jesus explains humility is necessary to become great (**Matthew 23:12**).

Discussion Questions

What is humility?

How does humility affect your life?

Why is humility important for childbirth?

Consider some common comments about childbirth. Do the comments represent pride, humility or giving up?

Add your personal insights

My Thoughts...

Accepting Your Adequacy

You have been created uniquely by God for the specific purposes to which he has called you. You have a unique collection of gifts, strengths, likes and abilities. You have been created for the work God determined for you before you were born. When you became a Christian, the Holy Spirit also bestowed upon you gifts for you to use in accomplishing the purposes God has for you.

Just as you have been uniquely created for a purpose, your child has also been created uniquely. From the start you will begin to recognize strengths, gifts, likes and abilities that are unique to this child. What is even more amazing is that God has chosen you to parent this child. Your motherhood is not an accident. You were selected to be the steward of this child of God. Though it may initially seem an impossible task, remember God does not give you a responsibility without making you adequate for the task.

Today, you may not feel ready to raise this son or daughter of God. If so, take a deep breath and remember all you are called to do today is to meet today's needs. As your child grows, so will you. Each milestone you mark for your child is also a milestone for you. Before long you will look back and wonder when it happened that you became so patient, or kind, or selfless, or giving, or honest, or loving. The truth is, your children will help you become the woman God created you to be and you will help your children prepare to fulfill the role God has set aside for them.

Letting Go

One of the most amazing things about giving birth is the way your body, the skin in which you live, directs the entire show. The uterus contracts, the cervix opens, the baby descends all without your brain deciding any of it needed to happen. You will not be in control. Labor may begin fast and hard, or labor may slowly build over a day or two. You may suddenly have a strong urge to push or you may slowly have a gentle urge to push. You do not get to choose.

What can be even your normal responses to the work your body is doing may not be considered polite. Some women fear behaving unacceptably during labor. You may get red in the face and your body may feel so hot you need to remove your clothing. You may vomit. You may poop. You may make the same faces and noises you make during sex.

The strong forces moving your baby into the world is your body, yet some women fear feeling helpless or powerless. Your eyes may close and you may not be able to tell people what you need or want. You may not even realize anyone else is in the room with you. That is real labor. But labor does not happen if you are not willing to give up control of your body for the few hours it takes to give birth.

What do you need to allow your body to do the things it needs to do to labor? How can you put aside your pride or need to control the image others have of you? What helps you trust that God made your body adequate to perform this work? Are you ready to let go of control long enough to let your body take over and welcome your child into this world?

48

Title: **Scripture Insight**

Page: 49

Type: Worksheet

Purpose: Explore scriptural concepts for pregnancy and birth

Time: 15 minutes or as homework

Discussion: Have the class review the verses, answering the questions. This can be done as a large group, while split into small groups or individually at home.

There are too many verses to have every verse read to every member of your class. There are several ways to approach the list in a manageable fashion. You may choose to use cards with the verses already written out; assign a few verses to each small group; or you may choose a small sample of the list encouraging further study at home.

The idea of birth being influenced by culture will be revisited in unit six, so do not feel you need to cover the entire topic at this point. It will be enough if the families begin to see that the people and events surrounding the new family do affect the birth.

The father may not specifically be mentioned. If families are familiar enough with the stories and characters, they can begin to draw conclusions from other verses around the birth.

The Bible was not written to record birth stories. It is a telling of the history of God working in the world. That makes it even more amazing that so many details about birth have been recorded.

Questions: What is most surprising about these birth stories in the Bible?

Pick one woman's story. In what ways can you relate to her story?

In what way are the births similar?

What can you pick out that is unique about each birth?

Scripture Insight

As you read through the following passages, pay attention to these questions:

1. What are the overall reactions to giving birth?
2. How is the greeting of a child influenced by culture and society?
3. How is the greeting of a child influenced by events in the mother's life?
4. What part does the father play in greeting the child?

Genesis 4:1-2
Genesis 4:1:17
Genesis 4:25
Genesis 16:15
Genesis 19:31-38
Genesis 21:1-5
Genesis 25:21-26
Genesis 29: 31-30:12
Genesis 30:21
Genesis 35:16-18
Genesis 38:27-30
Exodus 1:15-22
Exodus 2:14
Exodus 2:22
1 Chronicles 4:9
1 Samuel 1
1 Samuel 4:19
2 Samuel 12:15-24
Judges 13
Ruth 4:13
2 Kings 4:8-17
1 Samuel 4:19
Hosea 1
Matthew 1:18-25
Luke 1:57-58

To Pray About

In what ways do you fear you will fail as a parent?
In what ways do you feel prepared to parent?
What do you need to do to be ready to let go?

Unit Three
Greeting Baby

My Thoughts...

Unique Creations

Psalm 57:2

Psalm 139:14

John 19:25-27

Romans 12:6-8

Philippians 2:3-8

49

Overview

Making good decisions takes several key processes. First, you must understand what options are available. Then you must be able to accurately predict how those options will affect what is happening. Finally, you must be able to weigh the risks and benefits of each option to select the one most likely to produce the desired result.

As Christians, our definition of what constitutes a good decision is a little different from others. A good decision is not about bringing the most advantage to you. Instead, a good decision brings glory to God and demonstrates sacrificial love for others.

This unit requires several hours of research preparation for families. Be sure to introduce them to the information they need to explore before the class.

Unit Goals

After finishing the material in this unit, your students should be able to:

- List options available for giving birth
- Explain questions to ask before having an intervention
- List pros and cons of options for birth

Suggested Reading

Christian Childbirth Handbook

Options for Labor

Lord of Birth

Love

Birthing Naturally Web site

Options for birth (within Birth Planning)

Sample Schedule

Time	Activity	Page
15 Minutes	Options for Labor	52
30 Minutes	Pro and Con	53
20 Minutes	Making Decisions	54-55
30 Minutes	Case Studies	56-57
10 Minutes	Discussing Options	58-61

Overview

The options you have for labor will sometimes present themselves with a definite "answer." But just as frequently there will be no obvious right or wrong choice. It is the right and responsibility of the parents to make decisions that will affect the health of their child. You should never feel forced, coerced or manipulated into any decision.

When choosing how to handle labor, or when making any decision that will affect your child, a key point of stewardship will be loving your child with the sacrificial love Jesus modeled for us. Your decisions should be made focused on meeting the needs of and protecting your baby. This means your baby's health should be your highest priority.

There is no cookie cutter answer for what a labor should look like when the health of the baby is the highest priority. You will simply make the best decisions you can with the information you have at the time. That may mean you have exactly the birth you want, or you may not want the choices you know are right for labor.

Discussion Points

✓ There are a wide variety of options available for use as comfort measures that do not add risk for baby, and may actually help progress labor.

✓ Medicines are a tool. They are neither evil nor good. Depending on what is happening they can help or hinder you. Use them wisely.

✓ The attitude in which you make a decision may be more important than the decision you make. Whatever you decide to do, are you doing it out of a servant's heart?

✓ When seeking information, be sure to ask the question you want answered. A vague question will get a vague answer.

✓ Before you can build your birth plan, you will need to do some searching in your heart to discover what is most important for you.

Personal Study

✎ Ask some friends or relatives how they made their decisions about birth options. What sources of information did they use? In what ways were they satisfied? What would they change for their next labor, why?

✎ Read Bible stories that let you see an individual making decisions such as Cain (Genesis 4:1-16), Nehemiah (Nehemiah 1) or Daniel (Daniel 1). What good or bad patterns do you see?

✎ Make a list of questions to discuss with your doctor or midwife.

Unit Four
Choosing With Love

Scripture Checklist
❏ Luke 9:23-24
❏ 1 John 3:16
❏ Philippians 2:3-8
❏ John 13:34-35
❏ John 15:12
❏ 1 John 4:7-11
❏ Matthew 7:12
❏ Proverbs 14:8
❏ Psalm 20:4
❏ Proverbs 2:6
❏ Galatians 5:22
❏
❏
❏
❏

Suggested Readings
Lord of Birth
Love
Christian Childbirth Handbook
Options for Labor
Birthing Naturally Web site
Options for Childbirth

51

Title: **Options You May Have for Labor**

Page: 52

Type: Peer Teaching

Purpose: List available options for labor and birth.

Time: 15 minutes

Directions: This worksheet needs to be introduced to families before this class to give them time to investigate options.

              Ask families to get out their options sheet. Ask if there were any options they had trouble finding information about. Be sure to give other class members a chance to answer questions before answering them yourself.

              After questions are answered, ask families to volunteer to share two or three of the options they have selected and why. How do they expect this option to effect the course of labor?

Facilitating: Alternative presentation would be to show a birth video. Have families keep track of the options chosen by the woman in the video on the worksheet. After the movie is finished, have families share what they did or did not like.

              At this point you will want to begin the discussion about Biblical love. A list of questions about love is on page 63 of the student workbook. In pregnancy and childbirth, every decision you make can affect both the mother and the baby. Considering the potential effects to both helps ensure a good decision is made.

Materials: Birth Video

Scripture: John 13:34-35
              "A new command I give you: Love one another. As I have loved you, so you must love one another. By this all men will know that you are my disciples, if you love one another."

              Loving others was commanded by Jesus.

Unit Four
Choosing With Love
My Thoughts...

Options for Labor

Use this list to help you investigate your options and keep track of which ones are best for your labor. You do not need to include everything in a written birth plan; only include those issues about which you have a preference.

Starting or Speeding Labor
Spontaneous ○Up to 42 weeks ○Beyond 42 weeks
Self Induced ○Walk ○Enema ○Castor Oil ○Nipple Stimulation ○Acupressure
Medically Induced ○Prostaglandin Gel ○IV Oxytocin ○Amniotomy ○Misoprostol

Monitoring Labor
Intermittent ○Fetoscope ○Doptone ○External Monitor ○Telemetry
Continuous ○External Monitor ○Internal Monitor

Hydration
IV Fluids ○Saline Lock ○NPO (No liquids by mouth)
Clear Liquids ○Popsicles ○Ice Chips ○Lollipops ○Broth ○Tea ○Sodas
According to Thirst ○Limited to clear liquids ○No limit

Pain Relief
Relaxation Techniques ○Breathing ○Visualization ○Focus ○Massage ○Vocalization
Narcotic ○Only if requested ○Offer as soon as possible
Epidural/Spinal ○As Soon As Possible ○When Requested ○Walking/Light

Comfort Items and Techniques
Environment ○Lighting ○Temperature ○Music ○Fresh Air ○Own Clothing/Bedding
Water ○Labor Tub ○Birth Pool ○Shower
Massage Tools ○Tennis Ball ○Rolling Pin ○Heating Pad ○Ice Pack ○Lotion

Positions
Upright ○Walking ○Lunging ○Leaning on Wall/Person ○Sitting on Ball ○Rocking Chair
Hands and Knees ○With Ball ○On Bed ○Pelvic Rocking ○Chest to Floor
Reclining ○On side ○Recliner Chair

Pushing
Positions ○Squatting ○Standing ○Hands and Knees ○Reclining
Duration ○Spontaneous ○Directed ○Prolonged
Perineal Care ○Support ○Massage ○Compresses ○Positioning ○Episiotomy

Cesarean
Support ○Partner ○Doula ○Family Members
Anesthesia ○Epidural ○Spinal ○General
Environment ○Describe Events ○Video/Photos ○Baby and Mom Together for Recovery

Baby Care
Cord Cutting ○Partner ○Mother ○Family Members ○Wait until stops pulsing
Temperature Regulation ○Mother's Abdomen ○Warming Unit
Procedures ○Delay Procedures ○Vaccinations ○Circumcision ○First Bath ○Footprints
Nursery ○Rooming In ○Partner Rooming In ○Nursery on Request ○Pacifier / Bottle

Other options available at your birthplace:

52

Title: **Facing the Facts**

Page: 53

Type: Debate

Purpose: Demonstrate ability to discuss options for labor.

Time: 30 minutes

Directions: Allow the class to select two or three topics to investigate. Be sure the topic is related to labor and birth (i.e. not vaccinations or breast feeding) to ensure all families are properly prepared.

Split the class into two groups. One group will be "pro" the intervention (give reasons to use it in labor) while the other group is "con." Tell the groups to defend their position using the research they have gathered on the topic. Allow the pro group to go first with the con group providing rebuttals. Then let the con group present their arguments with the pro group giving rebuttals.

As the debate wears down, emphasize that families have demonstrated there are good and bad uses for the intervention discussed. Also point out that families are able to discuss research about options in an intelligent way

Facilitating: If you do not have information on interventions available for families, present this worksheet in the previous class to allow them time to do research.

If the families are not talkative or do not begin the debate on their own, ask questions about the intervention so they can answer from their assigned point of view. Examples of questions would be "under what circumstances should a woman be encouraged to have an elective cesarean."

The debates themselves will probably not last longer than 5 minutes each, but questions from families and discussion will continue. This is OK. The formal debate format may be intimidating to families, but it will force them to accept how much they do or do not know about options.

Materials: Intervention information sheets, books or pamphlets

My Thoughts...

Facing the Facts

There are many topics in the field of obstetrics that experts disagree about. To better understand some of the issues you face as a parent, choose a few topics that are important to you, and create a list of the pros and cons for those procedures or techniques. Some examples may be

Episiotomy
Elective Cesarean Section
Routine use of Electronic Fetal Monitors
Routine use of Intravenous Fluids
Oxytocin for labor augmentation or induction

You may find information in magazine articles, medical journals, newspapers, internet articles or books. As you review the literature, begin to think of questions you will want to ask of your health care professional. Also make sure you can answer questions such as:

• What is an appropriate use of the intervention?
• What are the risks of this intervention?
• What alternatives are available?
• How might this intervention be prevented?

Use this space to keep brief notes:

Topic:

Pro

Con

Topic:

Pro

Con

Topic:

Pro

Con

53

111

Title:	**Making Decisions About Interventions**
Page:	54
Type:	Fact Sheets
Purpose:	List the questions necessary for informed consent.
Time:	20 minutes
Directions:	Spend less than five minutes discussing the importance of each question. Split the class into small groups, or work as families. Give each group a labor decision card. Using the information they have researched, have the groups write out answers to each of the questions for the intervention suggested on the labor decision card..
	After five to ten minutes to seek the answers, have groups share their scenario and the information they found. Have them share any information they were unable to find. Have the class offer answers and suggestions of additional sources of information.
Facilitating:	Giving families time to work on the question before having them share increases the chance they will actually look up the information and participate in the discussion, but if time is tight, you could have the families work through a few scenarios as a large group.
	Activities that force families to use the information they are learning will do more to allow them to remember, understand and use the information when it comes time to make decisions in labor. If families need prompting, work through one scenario as a group.
Materials:	Intervention Information Sheets
Childbirth books
Labor Decision cards
Scripture:	Proverbs 2:6
For the LORD gives wisdom,
and from his mouth come knowledge and understanding.
	God can help you make a good decision even when you feel the options are overwhelming. God can give you wisdom even when you feel the choices are too complex.

My Thoughts...

Making Decisions About Interventions

Each intervention has specific benefits and risks. Most situations have more than one way you can handle them. Your job is to determine how to handle each situation so the benefits of your decision outweigh the risks.

What is the importance of knowing the answers to the following questions?

Why is this being recommended?

What do you hope will be accomplished by using this intervention?

What are the risks of using this intervention?

What is the next step if this does not work?

What are my other options and what are their risks?

Discussion Questions:
What are some ways to get the answers to these questions?
How do these ways compare to each other?

54

Title: **Handling Medication Side Effects**

Page: 55

Type: List making

Purpose: List ways to manage side effects of medications during labor.

Time: 5 minutes

Directions: Introduce this sheet after your families have identified some of the potential side effects of medications.

Introduce the suggestions listed on this worksheet as ways to manage the most common side effects for labor medications. These techniques can help if families decide medications are necessary for part of labor.

Remind families that not every woman has every side effect. Differences in timing of administration, position of baby, sensitivity to medications and specific medications used mean every woman will react to the medications in her own way. These are the most common reactions.

Facilitating: You may recommend families highlight the items they would like to have with them in their labor bag just in case.

Be sure families understand there is no way to predict side effects. These are possibilities if a medication is used and therefore should be considered as they evaluate the benefits and risks. However they will not know which side effects they will have until after the medication has been administered.

Previous experience with drugs, both prescription and street, may help predict side effects or outcomes with medications for labor. Encourage families to share medication histories with those helping them make drug-related decisions to have the best chance for the least side effects.

Materials: Bring as many items as possible to help demonstrate their use.

My Thoughts...

Handling Medication Side Effects

Although medications can help women during labor, they sometimes cause unwanted side effects. Not every woman will experience every side effect from a medication, and there is no way to know which side effects you may experience. For that reason, it is best to be familiar with a variety of ways to manage the most common side effects.

Itching

Cool cloths on skin
Cold packs on skin
Naloxone iv (reduces pain relief)
Avoid fentanyl in the next dose (reduces pain relief)
Diphenhydramine (makes you sleepy)

Shivering

Warm IV fluid
Warm blankets
Complete Relaxation/Hypnotic state

Nausea/Vomiting

Cool cloths or ice to forehead or neck
Peppermint lozenge
Peppermint, citrus or lavender essential oil
Fennel or ginger tea
Sugar water
Mouthwash
Pharmacological Relief

Urinary Retention

Empty bladder before administration
Try toilet/bedpan after 1 hour
Turn on trickling water
Be patient
Peppermint essential oil in the bedpan/toilet (1 drop)
Catheterization

Inadequate Pain Relief

Wait 20 minutes for full effect of medication
Turn to side of most pain (gravity helps)
Try to pinpoint where you feel pain
Call the anesthesiologist and explain what you feel
Use breathing and focusing techniques

Discussion Questions:

Which methods are most agreeable to you?
How can you be ready to use these during labor?

Title:	**Labor Stories One and Two**
Page:	56-57
Type:	Case Study
Purpose:	Predict appropriate uses of comfort measures, interventions and options available during labor.
Time:	30 minutes
Directions:	Have families read the case studies, either all together or in small groups. At the end are questions the groups should answer.
	Encourage families to think about options, comfort measures and interventions. How might labor have changed with the changes the families are making?
Facilitating:	Listen carefully as families share their thoughts and ideas. This activity is your opportunity to assess their understanding of the interventions. If they are using information wrong or making bad predictions, help them identify the correct way to use the information.
	Both stories use many interventions and have points where the mother was disappointed or did not get what she wanted. Take note of when these are brought up for the next activity.
	If families need more prompting, pass out comfort measure cards to help them identify additional options.
	Because these labor stories are written out with questions, you can choose a different labor story to present in class and assign these stories for homework. Additional activities for labor stories are on page 115.
Materials:	Comfort Measure cards.
Scripture:	Proverbs 14:8 The wisdom of the prudent is to give thought to their ways, but the folly of fools is deception.
	It is helpful to think about how we make decisions. In that way we can see what influences our decisions,. It is possible decisions have been made without realizing all the things to influence the decision.

My Thoughts...

Labor Story One

Read this story, paying attention to the choices made by the family. Answer the questions at the end of the story.

   I was on the phone with a friend after work when my water broke. No contractions, no sound, just suddenly sitting in a puddle of water. We quickly put our bags in the car and my husband drove to the hospital.

   I had changed clothes before we left, but was soaked again by the time we arrived at the hospital. After I got into the bed, the nurse attached a monitor and asked me the standard questions. I still had no contractions.

   Our doctor came by to see me around 9:00 p.m. When he checked, I was two to three centimeters dilated but still not having any contractions. The doctor knew we wanted a natural birth, so recommended I walk around to see if labor would start. I walked around for two hours and still had no contractions. My doctor came back to discuss some blood work with me. He informed me the results meant I should be induced now instead of waiting for labor to start on its own.

   The nurse attached IV synthetic oxytocin, and within five minutes I had very painful contractions. I used the breathing and relaxation techniques I had learned until 4:30 in the morning when I asked for some pain medication. The nurse checked me before giving me a narcotic, and I was 4 centimeters.

   The narcotic made me feel drunk but was not doing anything for the pain I felt. The nurse checked me again at 6:30, I was 8 centimeters that time. She said if I wanted an epidural I needed to have one now or it would be too late. I told her no, and was upset that she would say that to me.

   I felt the urge to push by 7:30. The nurse checked me, and I was fully dilated. I pushed as hard as I could, and my baby was born at 9:10.

1. Where might you have made the same decisions?

2. Where might you have made different decisions?

3. What are possible outcomes of decisions you would make?

4. What other options are available, even if you would not choose them?

5. What are the possible outcomes of the other options?

56

Instructions for **Case Studies** is on the previous page.

Additional ways to use labor stories

Find a few labor stories that give details of how mom was feeling, and rewrite them removing mention of comfort measures used. Pass out comfort measure cards to families. As you read the story, pause when appropriate and ask families if any of their comfort measures would be helpful at this point in labor.

Retype a labor story separating the obvious stages of labor onto individual cards. If enough detail is given, separate the various stages into two or three cards each. Ask families to read the labor story, have them place the sections of the story into groups according to stage of labor. To make this more challenging, do not indicate on the cards which order they should be read.

Print out copies of the labor clock. As you read a labor story to the group, ask them to pay attention to what the mother is feeling and/or what comfort measures are used. After the story is read, have the families create a labor clock representing the labor in the story.

For a more advanced class, ask the class to diagram a labor story. This means they will visually represent the circumstances and decisions that are inter-related. It may look like a webbing diagram, a decision tree or any other diagram format the class is most comfortable with. The idea is to give them the opportunity to see how the decisions and outcomes are related.

Allow your class the freedom to rewrite a labor story. Read the story through once so families can get an understanding of the circumstances of the labor. As you read through again, have families change the way the mother responds to labor. This may mean using different comfort measures or different decisions. Keep the main circumstances the same—if the mother in the story had a cesarean, she will still have a cesarean. Ask the families how their reactions to the story change with their changes, even with the same results.

Rewrite a labor story taking out all indicators of how long the labor is. Remove all time references and change comments such as "a few hours" to "later." Read the story to your families. Ask them to share their initial reactions to the labor. Then ask them how long they thought it lasted. Tell them how long the labor actually lasted, then ask them if knowing the length changed their reaction to the labor story.

Rewrite a labor story removing all mention of how the mother is feeling. Leave in the length of labor and the decisions she made. Read the story to your families. Ask them to share their initial reactions to the labor. Families will be amazed by how differently they interpreted the same events. This can help families understand how individually they need to approach labor preparation.

My Thoughts...

Labor Story Two

Read this story, paying attention to the choices made by the family. Answer the questions at the end of the story.

I just expected my baby was going to be born on my due date. But the due date came and went without any signs of labor. A week after my due date I was a physical and emotional wreck. I could not believe how much weight I had gained, my whole body felt swollen, I could not wear my shoes. I broke down and cried to my doctor, so he decided I should be induced.

I arrived at the hospital at 6:00 am, filled out the paperwork and was officially admitted by 8:00. As part of the admitting, a nurse anesthetist came to explain the pain medication options to me. I was very opposed to anyone putting a needle in my back, and how bad could labor be anyway?

My induction started around 9, and my water was spontaneously broken by 10. I just remember the contractions being so strong and the pressure being severe. I would walk back and forth between the bathroom and the bed, dragging the IV with me.

By 11 I was in tears, begging for an epidural. The nurse told me I could not have an epidural until I was 4 centimeters. As I was trying to convince her to check my dilation, I started to have an urge to push. She seemed shocked and quickly checked me. She felt my baby's head and called for my doctor. She gave me a shot to help me relax, which I thought was wonderful. My baby was born at 12:30.

1. What evidence can you see that tells you this might be a fast labor?

2. Can you identify the stages of labor for this mother?

3. What options did this woman choose to use?

4. What options were available to this woman that she did not use?

5. What effects might those options have had?

6. Where might you have made different decisions?

57

Title: **Discussing Options with your Caregiver**

Page: 58

Type: Discussion

Purpose: Identify strategies for discussing choices with caregivers.

Time: 10 minutes

Directions: Introduce the page to families. Explain they will want to start talking about birth issues with their caregiver. List the steps for having a good discussion as

1) Plan (write out questions and inform caregiver of desire to talk);

2) Discuss (actually talking to and listening to responses of the caregiver); and

3) Review (collecting additional information to further discuss or decide to change caregivers)

They will repeat these steps several times before they have a final birth plan.

Ask families to come up with wording for questions to obtain information from their caregiver.

Facilitating: The episiotomy questions are given as an example. Choose a topic that has been important to families over the class and let them come up with questions for that topic. For example, with synthetic oxytocin "what methods to induce labor will you try before using synthetic oxytocin?" or "what would make you think synthetic oxytocin should not be used?"

An alternate presentation would be to make a game. Split the room into work groups and pass out identical caregiver discussion scenario cards to each group. Ask the groups to write a question to ask for each scenario. Have the groups share their question and vote on the best wording.

Materials: Discussion Cards

Scripture: Matthew 7:12
So in everything, do to others what you would have them do to you, for this sums up the Law and the Prophets.

It can be difficult to deal with a health care provider when you feel they are disrespecting you, however we are called to treat even our enemies with love. This does not mean you need to continue to work with a provider you disagree with. If you feel the need to leave a provider, be kind but firm.

Discussing Options with your Caregiver

Some women get nervous when they talk to their caregiver. This nervousness is unnecessary. Your caregiver is working for you. If you are dissatisfied with the quality of work she is doing for you, hire someone else.

Plan

✓ Research the topics that are most important to you.

✓ Keep a list of questions and issues you want to discuss with your caregiver. Take it with you to your appointments so you do not forget anything.

Discuss

✓ Let your caregiver know at the beginning of the appointment that you want to ask a few questions; if she forgets, gently remind her before the appointment is done. Be sure to let your caregiver know you are interested in her thoughts and opinions of the options in general and in your case specifically.

✓ When possible take something you have read on the subject with you. Share with your caregiver the sources of information you have on the subject and why they have led you to the conclusions you have made.

✓ Ask your caregiver if she has any literature on the subject, or if she can recommend a book or web site so you can keep researching the issue. If your caregiver disagrees with your views on a subject, let her know you will continue to research the subject and want to talk to her about it again at your next appointment. This will give her time to do some more research and gather information to help you make a decision. It also lets her know that this issue is important to you.

Review

✓ Consider the information you received from your caregiver and any new research she suggested.

✓ Maintain a list of questions and ideas to share at your next appointment.

How to Ask Questions

When asking questions, ask the specific questions you want the answered. Asking, "How often do you do episiotomies?" will give you the answer, "I only do them when necessary." Instead ask,

"How many of your clients need episiotomies?"
"Under what circumstances do you recommend an episiotomy?"
"What techniques do you use to help keep perineal skin intact?"

Write three questions you will ask of your caregiver at your next visit.

1.

2.

3.

58

121

Title:	**My Choices**
Page:	59
Type:	List Making
Purpose:	Identify preferred options.
Time:	Less than 10 minutes

Directions: Explain that all families have an ideal birth, and they all have ideas about what choices they would and would not like. Some families are concerned about writing their choices because they believe it makes them seem inflexible or difficult to work with. Other families have been told people who write birth plans always have cesareans.

The truth is, not writing out or discussing your choices will not make your hopes and desires for this birth go away. Instead, by not sharing your desires for this birth with your caregivers you increase the chances you will not have the birth you want.

Introduce this page to your families, explaining this is the first step in writing a birth plan. Give families time to finish each sentence. If the group is willing, have them share their answers.

Sharing answers gives the families practice discussing their options. The most important question is number five. If time is an issue for your group, focus on this question.

Facilitating: This is the first step in birth planning. Some families will be beyond this step while others will be nervous they are not giving the "right" answers. Stress that there is no perfect birth plan, and there is no right or wrong on a birth plan. The only way to make a mistake is to not be honest about how you would like to handle labor.

If there is no time in class, or if families are not yet ready to answer these questions, this worksheet can be completed as homework.

Scripture: Psalm 20:4
May he give you the desire of your heart
and make all your plans succeed.

God is in control of labor, but that does not mean he is unconcerned with your desires. God can give you the labor you hope for.

Workbook Page 59

My Thoughts...

My choices

You have explored the normal process of labor, comfort measures and the options available. You have probably begun making decisions about how you want to handle labor. Complete these statements.

1. If everything goes perfect, I would like my labor to be...

2. If safety concerns arise before labor begins, I would like to...

3. If safety concerns arise during labor, I would like to...

4. If my comfort plan is inadequate during labor, I would like to...

5. To increase my chances of having the labor I desire, I am...

59

123

Title:	**Epidural Assessment**
Page:	60
Type:	Questioning
Purpose:	Identify misunderstandings about epidurals.
Time:	5 to 10 minutes
Directions:	Families can complete this assessment in class or at home. After completing the assessment, discuss any questions which are interesting or surprised the families.
Facilitating:	All odd questions are false. All even questions are true. Student Workbooks give this answer on page 62. Discussion for each question is on the teacher web site. Familiarize yourself with the discussion of each question to save time looking for answers during class.

Answers to these questions are in general. It is possible to have an epidural and have labor suddenly move fast. It is possible to have a faulty administration of an epidural and have a headache. The answers are based on research evidence. Try to avoid getting bogged down into discussions of personal experience that are contrary to research unless the class has a good understanding of statistics.

If you are working with a class who misunderstood epidurals, be prepared for questions and disagreement. Many women are given inaccurate information about this technique. Some families in your class may have made decisions based on misinformation believing they were doing the best for labor. Learning the truth can be traumatic. If this happens, remain calm. Remind families epidural is a tool, and like any other tool it has good and bad uses. The goal here is to understand epidurals so you can better discern the difference between a good and bad use.

When working with experienced mothers be alert for mothers who devalue the decisions they made during previous labors. Remind families they made the best decisions with the information they had at the time. It is not fair to compare past decisions with current knowledge. We are all growing and learning. They are now educated and can make a better decision next time.

My Thoughts...

Epidural Assessment

Mark each statement as true or false, then turn to page 62 to check your answers.

1. An epidural removes the pain while allowing labor to continue normally.

2. Epidurals are the most effective medications for managing pain during labor.

3. An epidural will remove all the pain of labor.

4. It may take up to an hour to receive relief after choosing to have an epidural.

5. You can still walk with an epidural.

6. An epidural can allow a woman to sleep during labor.

7. Epidurals do not affect the baby.

8. Epidural administration requires you to sit still even during contractions.

9. Epidurals improve satisfaction with labor.

10. Epidurals are not always readily available.

11. There is a cut-off after which you will not be allowed to have an epidural.

12. You can have an epidural with a midwife.

13. You need to stop an epidural for pushing.

14. Epidurals are used for cesarean surgical births.

15. Epidurals reduce the chances you will tear or need an episiotomy.

16. An epidural can affect your baby's heart rate.

17. Epidurals speed labor.

18. Women with epidurals often need a catheter to urinate.

19. Epidurals do not increase the rate of cesarean surgery.

20. There is no standard dosage/technique for epidural medication use during labor.

21. Epidurals cause headaches.

22. Epidurals require continuous fetal monitoring.

23. There are no side effects with epidural.

24. Women with an epidural need to change positions regularly to prevent a "window" of pain on one side.

25. You cannot use an epidural if you have had a previous cesarean.

Title:	**What Will I Choose?**
Page:	61
Type:	Reflection
Purpose:	Application of scripture to personal birth preparation.
Time:	Less than 5 minutes.
Directions:	Explain to families this is an interpretation of Galatians 5:22-23, commonly referred to as the fruit of the Spirit. Read it aloud as a class, giving each family a different section to read.
	Remind families this was just one person's interpretation of how to live out the fruits of the Spirit in labor. Invite them to share how they would live out this scripture.
	Encourage families to rewrite this verse on their own to reflect their interpretation and the way they would express the fruits of the Spirit.
Facilitating:	As an example of different ways to interpret the verse, one family may interpret kindness to mean the mother should not scream at the people trying to help her. Another family may interpret kindness to mean the father should remain with the mother to meet her needs.
	If the class has a way to share, they may enjoy reading other families interpretations. This can easily be done by bringing a printed copy to class, e-mailing copies or using a class web group.
Scripture:	Galatians 5:22-23 But the fruit of the Spirit is love, joy, peace, patience, kindness, goodness, faithfulness, gentleness and self-control. Against such things there is no law.

Workbook Page 61

My Thoughts...

What Will I Choose?

I have a choice to make. For the next few hours I will be engaged in the most demanding work I have ever done. But since this is the most important work I will ever do…

I will do it with love…
This is my baby's birth day. It is not about my needs, my desires, my hopes or my feelings. Because I love my child, I will put myself in God's hands so I can concentrate on giving my baby the birth he needs.

I will do it with joy…
Although I may feel temptation to wallow in self-pity, I will be thankful for every contraction. I will rejoice that every contraction brings me one step closer to the moment I have waited for so long.

I will do it with peace…
I will not battle my body or my baby. I will simply allow my baby to use my body as an entrance point for life.

I will do it with patience…
I will not lose sight of the fact that my sense of time may be skewed, and what feels like a lifetime is really only a few hours of waiting. I will not make decisions that put myself or my baby at risk simply to shorten the time I must wait.

I will do it with kindness…
I will be kind to my baby; she is alone, and she may be frightened. I will not allow myself to benefit by putting her at risk.

I will do it with goodness…
I will not let myself give into the temptation to use labor as an excuse to be rude, angry, mean, hurtful, lazy or prideful. This is my first opportunity to teach my baby about relationships.

I will do it with faithfulness…
I will not question God's love or goodness as I pass through this time of trial. I will not let my actions or reactions be a reason for others to question my love or goodness.

I will do it with gentleness…
As I welcome my baby, may he only hear my voice raised in joy; may she only see my arms raised in praise; and may he only feel the touch of love.

I will do it with self control…
I will not allow myself to lower my standards simply because I am in labor. I will continue to strive for excellent character regardless of the challenges.

In a few moments, my baby will arrive. For the next few hours, I will be exposed to labor's demands. It is now that I must make a choice.

Discussion Question:
How would you interpret Galatians 5:22-23?

Workbook Page 62 contains two devotional thoughts families can read.

Notes on **Scripture Checklist** from page 51

One of the first lessons many Christians learn is the need to give up one's own ambitions to follow Christ (**Luke 9:23-24**). This is as true in labor as any other part of life. Personal ambition should be set aside when making decisions. Personal ambition may include wanting others to accept or think highly of the mother. Personal ambition may also be having the easiest or most comfortable labor.

Once personal ambitions are set aside, you are free to make decisions based on love. We are commanded to love others (**John 13:24-25; John 15:12; 1 John 4:7-11**). Jesus said to love God and love others was the most important commandment (**Matthew 7:12; Matthew 22:36-40**). Unfortunately, love is often a misunderstood concept. What does Biblical love look like? Biblical love is displayed in actions (**Philippians 2:3-8**). Biblical love lays itself down for others (**1 John 3:16**).

As we consider the decisions we make for labor, we must determine if our decisions have been made from love (**Proverbs 14:8**). The goal cannot be the image of a perfect birth, instead the goal needs to be a healthy mother and healthy baby. It is possible to achieve that goal with the perfect birth, but achieving that perfect birth is not the first priority.

Making wise decisions does not mean you must suffer and hate labor. God can give you the desires of your heart (**Psalm 20:4**). The problem arises when our desires are opposed to him.

Discussion Questions

What are common priorities for labor planning?

Do these priorities reflect love?

What might labor look like if the goal was Biblical love?

How can you be sure your decisions are made in love?

Add your personal insights

My Thoughts...

Hearing the Voice of God

Sometimes the voice of God is as loud as the thunder, you know clearly what you should do. Sometimes the voice of God is as soft as a gentle breeze; unless you quiet yourself and listen, you will not hear it. If you are not sure where God is leading you for this birth, consider trying a new way to listen for his voice. There are as many ways to quiet yourself before God as there are unique people he has created.

You could go for a walk in the woods, on the beach, through the fields, up a mountain or in the heart of the city.

You could sit silently under a tree, at the edge of the ocean, in a crowded coffee shop or your own bedroom.

You might need to stop working through your to-do list, or begin a project you have been putting off.

You might want to open your mouth to pour out your heart, keep your mouth closed for a while or use your voice to sing worship and praise.

You may need to begin letting others serve you, or begin serving others.

You may want to read a different version of the Bible or listen to a recorded Bible.

Explore new ways to spend time with God. Enjoy yourself as you learn about all the unique voices he uses to speak with you.

Making Good Use of Your Tools

Medicine and other health technology are tools. They are neither good nor evil. Depending on how labor is progressing, they can either help or hinder the process. Use them wisely.

The key to making good use of your tools is to be aware of the risks and benefits. Using a tool that adds minimal benefit while increasing risk to you or your baby is unwise. At best, tools should be used to decrease the risk, at minimum they should not add risk.

In general, there is more than one way to handle any labor challenge. A tired mother may benefit from a narcotic, but she may also benefit from a massage, a warm bath, changing positions or deep relaxation between contractions. Once you know what tools may be beneficial, you can look at the associated risks.

One way to maintain the lowest risk possible is to always use the tools with the lowest risk first. If that does not work, you can always try something with more risk. Give yourself adequate time to try low-risk tools before moving on to higher risk tools. Your goal should always be to keep the risk as low as possible for both you and your baby.

Epidural Assessment:

All the even numbered questions are true. All the odd numbered statements are false. For more information about epidural pain relief for labor, please see the Birthing Naturally web site at www.birthingnaturally.net.

Title:	**Scripture Insight**
Page:	63
Type:	Discussion
Purpose:	Explore scriptural concepts for pregnancy and birth
Time:	15 minutes or as homework
Discussion:	Have the class review the verses, answering the questions. This can be done as a large group, while split into small groups or individually at home.

Love can be a difficult concept to grasp, especially in a world that defines love by candy, cards, roses and romance movies. Giving families time to discuss what love is, and what love is not can help them see changes that may need to be made in their life.

Biblical love is sacrificial. It is laying down your life for another. It is making the needs of others a higher priority than yourself. And though we generally consider the need to love others when we think about our enemies, we must also practice sacrificial love for those close to us.

There is no right answer for what a labor looks like when decisions are made in love. It simply means decisions are made to reduce risk for the baby and the mother; not for convenience or to achieve the "right" experience.

Questions: What are reasons (good and bad) families make decisions in labor?

What does it mean to make a decision in love?

What might it mean to lay down your life for someone? What might it mean to lay down your life for your child in labor?

Workbook Page 63

Scripture Insight

As you read through the verses from the scripture checklist on page 51, meditate on these questions.

1. What does it mean that God loves you?

2. What does it mean to love God?

3. Explain why Christ is our example of love.

4. Describe what life is like when loving God is your first priority.

5. In what ways do you feel pregnancy can display your love for God?

6. In what ways do you feel giving birth can display your love for God?

To Pray About

In the past, how have you been sure you are following God's plan?
What options for labor do you feel uncomfortable about? Why?
Seek the wisdom of God for making decisions.

My Thoughts...

Wisdom

Proverbs 2:6

Proverbs 16:3

Psalm 119:148

Isaiah 58:11

1 Timothy 4:14

Overview

We sometimes get this idea in our head that labor becomes more difficult linearly. In other words, the longer a woman is in labor the more difficult labor becomes. While this may be true for some women, there is no way to predict what will be the hardest part of labor.

Transient internal events such as a full bladder, position of the baby, mother's fatigue or dehydration in the mother can cause a sudden increase in discomfort. Similarly external events such as the laboring environment, changing locations or lack of emotional support can cause a challenge. If the situation is resolved, the labor may become less difficult.

Other events may cause a more enduring labor challenge or a labor emergency. During these times, options may be limited and stress levels may be high. It is important to understand what options may be available when labor does not go as planned. To know their options, families must learn how to tell the difference between a normal variation of labor, a variation that indicates a potential problem and a birth emergency.

There are two parts to overcoming a labor challenge. The first is physical; identify appropriate reactions, make changes to the labor and hopefully have the challenge resolved. The second is spiritual; ensure the challenge does not interfere with your faith and trust in God as Lord.

Unit Goals

After finishing the material in this unit, your students should be able to:

- List common challenges and difficulties of labor.
- Explain possible ways of handling challenges or difficult labors.
- Describe the options available for surgical birth.

Suggested Reading

Christian Childbirth Handbook

Labor Challenges

Lord of Birth

Faith

Birthing Naturally Web site

Labor Challenges

Sample Schedule

Time	Activity	Page
15 Minutes	Difficult Spots in Labor	66
30 Minutes	Variations and Emergencies	67
20 Minutes	Handling Labor Challenges	69-70
20 Minutes	Labor Challenges Role Play	71

Overview

The truth is sometimes hard to see. How can you be sure that what you are deciding is the best option unless you understand the truth about what is happening? There are many variations of the normal, healthy labor. You may be experiencing something that is not average, and still be completely healthy. Knowing what signals a problem and being able to adjust for that problem are key components of stewardship.

There are several ways in which you may be challenged during labor. It is not enough to just recognize the challenge; you will need to be able to respond to the challenge effectively. The goal of this unit is to learn to differentiate between a birth emergency and a normal variation of labor; and how to respond to each.

While preparing to make wise decisions, it is possible to over-prepare. Birth emergencies are very rare, so your chances of experiencing one are small. It is possible to struggle with trusting God instead of your knowledge. Not only should you aim to make good decisions during a challenge, but also to continue experiencing the peace of God during the storm.

Discussion Points

✓ Some challenges will present themselves before labor begins, giving you a chance to make changes during pregnancy.

✓ Using medical interventions when a challenge arises will make changes. Sometimes the changes are what you want, and other times they are not.

✓ God has a purpose for your labor, and he will teach you something from labor. However, you may not discover what it is until months later.

✓ Even if you make changes, you may not be able to end a labor challenge. You can only respond to what is happening; you cannot control your labor.

✓ There are a number of reasons why a woman may experience a challenge in labor. It is not necessarily a sign of a lack of faith.

Personal Study

✎ Make a list of your gifts and strengths. How can you use those to overcome any challenges?

✎ Talk to family and friends about their labor and birth challenges. What options did they choose? How did those options change labor?

✎ Reread the story of your favorite Bible character. What can you learn from the stories of challenges in the Bible?

Unit Five
Labor Challenges

Scripture Checklist
❑ Isaiah 55:8-9
❑ Proverbs 18:13
❑ John 8:32
❑ James 3:17
❑ John 14:27
❑ James 1:2-4
❑ Psalm 4:8
❑ Psalm 29:11
❑ Deuteronomy 31:6
❑
❑
❑
❑

Suggested Readings

Lord of Birth
Faith

Christian Childbirth Handbook
Labor Challenges

Birthing Naturally Web site
Labor Challenges

65

Title:	**Difficult Spots in Labor**
Page:	66
Type:	Brainstorming
Purpose:	Identify difficult times in labor; list ways to manage them.
Time:	5 to 10 minutes
Directions:	Explain there are normal times of increased stress in labor when it may become more difficult to manage the discomfort. These times are listed on the worksheet.
	Ask families to share ideas about why these times become more difficult. Is the stress inevitable? What can families do to prepare for these times in labor so they are not overpowering? What can families do during labor if they experience difficulties during these times?
	Let families know this list is not complete. Other difficult spots in labor include any time the mother has a full bladder, when the mother is dehydrated or if the mother is in an uncomfortable position. In some instances, a quick response can significantly decrease the discomfort and difficulty of labor.
Facilitating:	Use this opening discussion to begin talking about the differences between the way the world "overcomes" trials and the way a Christian "overcomes" trials.
	You may want to use one or more of the following questions to begin this discussion.
	Does trusting God mean you will never have trouble?
	Does God promise us whatever we ask for?
	Should God be required to give us everything we want?
Scripture:	Isaiah 55:8-9 "For my thoughts are not your thoughts, neither are your ways my ways," declares the LORD.
	"As the heavens are higher than the earth, so are my ways higher than your ways and my thoughts than your thoughts.
	It takes humility to accept that you do not understand everything about labor. God had a plan when he designed the labor process, and he has a plan as he orchestrates each baby's entrance to the world.
	God demonstrates great creativity in the variety of reproduction methods in the plant and animal worlds. Encourage families to consider some of the reasons God may have created human labor as he did.

Unit Five
Labor Challenges
My Thoughts...

Difficult Spots in Labor

You can expect there will be certain times during labor that will be more difficult than others. Be prepared to handle these occurrences.

Why might the following times be difficult?
What could be done to help the mother through this difficult spot?

Onset of labor

Moving to the hospital

During examination

Beginning of transition

Beginning of pushing

Crowning

Discussion Question:
What does it mean to persevere through a trial?
How do you, as a Christian, overcome a challenge?

66

Title:	**Variations of Normal & Birth Emergencies**
Page:	67-68
Type:	Lecture
Purpose:	List problems that may occur during labor.
Time:	20 minutes
Directions:	Work through the outline on the worksheet to explain the challenges before and during labor. Explain if and why these challenges may be a problem and allow families to make recommendations for ways to manage these situations.
	Explain how to manage a birth emergency and how to obtain help as fast as possible in your area.
Facilitating:	If families have experience with labor, they may choose to share about these topics. Be sure to balance their need to share with keeping a schedule.
	Families may begin to feel unnecessarily nervous. Stress how common or how rare each of the variations are. Be sure to explain what the perceived danger is in each instance, and what families can do about each one.
Materials:	Variations Cheat Sheet
Scripture:	Psalm 4:8 I will lie down and sleep in peace, for you alone, O LORD, make me dwell in safety.
	Psalm 29:11 The LORD gives strength to his people; the LORD blesses his people with peace.
	It is possible to have peace in the midst of a labor challenge. God can keep you safe. God can give you strength.

Workbook Page 67

Variations of Normal Before Labor

You may know about some challenges before labor begins, allowing you time to make changes.

What is challenging in each of these situations?
Which challenges are you facing?
What options do you have for managing your challenges?

Breech Position

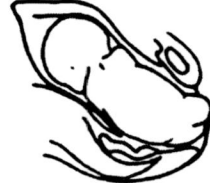

Transverse Position

Gestational Diabetes

Group B Strep

Overdue/ Postmaturity

History of Abuse

Advanced Maternal Age

Sixth or more time giving birth

Multiple Pregnancy

Pre-eclampsia

Obesity

Unit Five
Labor Challenges
My Thoughts...

67

Instructions for **Variations of Normal** is on the previous page.

Spiritual challenges for mothers

In addition to the regular challenges for labor, mothers with a previous traumatic birth experience or attempting a VBAC may find themselves working through the challenges from their previous labor. This increases the stress during labor which may hinder attempts to labor normally.

Of equal concern for the Christian mother is the condition of the mother's heart after a traumatic birth experience. Be aware that people deal with hurt in different ways. Some ways lead to healing, others lead to bitterness. Some ways help the mother find her strength, others leave a mother feeling helpless or worthless. As you help the family prepare for the upcoming birth, you may need to spend time helping them heal from the wounds of births past.

If possible, place mothers with spiritual challenges together in a separate class. This will allow you to spend less time on basics of pregnancy so you can devote more time to healing.

Give families adequate time to share their story. Acknowledge their hurts without trying to fix the problem for them. Remember God can heal their wounds, you cannot. Help them seek healing by spending time with them in prayer.

If a family is struggling with bitterness, gently encourage them as they learn to forgive the individuals they blame for their bad labor experience.

As they plan for the upcoming birth, encourage families to share about what worked, and what did not work for them in labor. Though the experience did not turn out how they expected, they have become experts on how they would like to handle labor.

Some families will have already begun to research what they "did wrong" last time. Remind families that they made the best decision with the information they had at the time. Judging their decisions from a past birth based on what they know now (including how the labor unfolded) is unfair. Instead, they should focus on using the additional knowledge they have gained to be better prepared for the upcoming labor.

In some families, bitterness or worthlessness in respect to labor gets passed down from mother to daughter. When possible, allow families to share what they learned about birth as they were growing up.

Above all, help families understand the outcome of a birth experience is not a legitimate test for their faithfulness or God's love. God loves them, and God can allow them to have a challenging labor. A woman can have strong faith and experience a challenging labor.

Workbook Page 68

Unit Five
Labor Challenges

My Thoughts...

Variations of Normal During Labor

Some challenges you will not know about until labor begins. What are these challenges, and what options do you have if they occur?

Discouraged Mother

Fast Labor

Posterior Baby

Ascynclitic Baby

Premature Rupture of Membranes

Slow Progress

Birth Emergencies

A birth emergency is not a normal variation of labor. It is an emergency situation in which your baby's life is in danger. True birth emergencies are rare. What are each of these emergencies, and what can be done about them?

Fetal Distress

Placental Previa

Placental Abruption

Umbilical Cord Prolapse

Hemorrhage

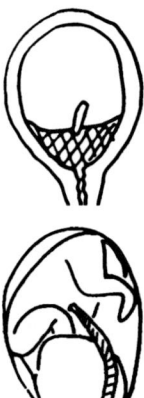

68

139

Title:	**Handling Labor Challenges**
Page:	69
Type:	List Making
Purpose:	Identify appropriate responses to labor challenges.
Time:	15 minutes
Directions:	The Venn diagram should be filled out by families. This can be done individually or as a group with one diagram being completed on a dry erase board.
	Select one normal and one dangerous variation. Write these in the appropriate circle of the diagram. Some variations may be normal and signal a potential for danger. These can be placed in the space between the two circles.
	Have families choose a comfort measure, position change or intervention that may be used for both the normal and dangerous challenge. Write this in the response section of the diagram.
	Ask families to think about what potential outcomes may occur if the intervention is used in response to the dangerous variation. Write the outcomes in the overlapping space between response and dangerous. Now do the same for the normal category.
	What you really want families to grasp at this point is that one intervention may help prevent problems or add more problems. If families begin to understand this point, they can begin to see the importance of determining what is happening and making a wise decision.
	Point out that sometimes it is difficult to tell what is causing the problem. For example, slow labor may be caused by many things. If you do not know what is causing it, what effect can an intervention have on your labor? How might a family approach such a problem?
Facilitating:	Attempting to diagram every labor challenge can be confusing. Have families start with one challenge, adding more if time allows.
Materials:	Dry erase board and markers
Scripture:	John 8:32
Then you will know the truth, and the truth will set you free.
	Understanding the truth about labor challenges sets us free from unnecessary worry and fear. Understanding the ways interventions can affect labor sets us free from second guessing our decisions later.

Workbook Page 69

My Thoughts...

Handling Labor Challenges

Knowing how to handle a labor challenge requires understanding what is happening, and how your body may react to the various options. To help you organize this information, take some time to make a Venn diagram.

1. Determine if what is happening is a normal variation of labor, is a variation that may signal a potential complication, or is a dangerous situation for mother and/or baby. Place the challenges in the appropriate part of the diagram.

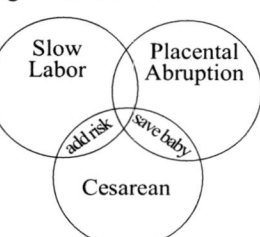

2. Select a response to the challenge, such as induction, position change or surgical birth. Place the response in the appropriate part of the diagram.

3. In the overlap between response and challenges, write what you may expect from using this response in this situation.

Discussion Question:
Why is it important to understand the potential effects of the options for responding to labor challenges?

69

141

Title: **Cesarean Surgery**

Page: 70

Type: Lecture

Purpose: List options available for a cesarean birth.

Time: 10 minutes

Directions: Have families share ideas about why a woman may need a cesarean birth. This may include reasons they have heard from friends and family or things they have read. Be sure to answer any questions and correct any misunderstandings.

                     Describe the procedure for a cesarean completely. Then return to the procedure and explain options families may have.

Facilitating: Stress that the options for a cesarean are different if the surgery is planned before labor begins. However, women who select cesarean for birth to respond to a challenge in labor do still have options.

                     You may find a short video of a cesarean helpful for families to understand the process.

                     Families not planning a cesarean may be hesitant to consider their options. Remind families that in an emergency situation, they will not have time to consider the options available. Making decisions now can help increase their satisfaction if a cesarean is necessary.

                     Understand the influence of culture on your ability to present this topic. Some cultures believe words cause events. This means if they talk openly about having a cesarean, they will have a cesarean. Do not force conversations about what specific families would do if you suspect this. Instead, present the topic by saying, "We all know someone who has had a cesarean. I want to be sure we understand the differences between a cesarean and vaginal birth."

Scripture: Deuteronomy 31:6
                     Be strong and courageous. Do not be afraid or terrified because of them, for the LORD your God goes with you; he will never leave you nor forsake you.

                     Having an unplanned cesarean surgery does not mean failure, and it does not mean God has left you. God stays with you through all challenges in your life.

Unit Five
Labor Challenges
My Thoughts...

Cesarean Surgery

Some reasons for cesarean birth include...

If a cesarean is done, these procedures will happen...

If a cesarean is done, these procedures might happen...

If a cesarean is done, these options may be available. Talk to your doctor or midwife to find out what additional options are available.

When to start the surgery

When to have family join you

Medication used

Support person with you at all times

Photo or video documentation

Surgeon describes events

Immediate breast feeding

Someone with baby at all times

70

Title:	**Labor Challenges Role Play**
Page:	71
Type:	Problem Solving
Purpose:	Identify appropriate responses to labor challenges.
Time:	20 minutes
Directions:	If the class is large, split into smaller groups. Give each group two or three scenarios and allow them time to discuss the options available. After a few minutes, have the groups come back together and share their ideas.
	If the class is small enough, work through all the labor challenges as a group. You can either read the scenarios yourself allowing anyone to comment, or you can assign each family a scenario to read and make first comments. If you assign scenarios, give families a minute or two to review their scenario and collect their thoughts before asking them to read and share ideas.
Facilitating:	This worksheet can be done in class as small groups, or completed at home. Be aware that some families may not complete it at home, but may still be willing to participate in the discussion about it.
	To assign as homework, ask families to complete this worksheet at home. At the next class, ask them to share any areas they had concerns about or could not find answers for. Ask them to share the answers they found.
	Additional discussion question, "What can you do now to reduce the likelihood of this challenge?"
Scripture:	Proverbs 18:13 He who answers before listening—that is his folly and his shame.
	To make wise decisions during a labor challenge, you must first understand what the challenge is.

Workbook Page 71

My Thoughts...

Labor Challenges Role Play

How might a mother handle the following challenging labor situations?

Mother appears to be in early labor. She is not using any comfort measures yet, can still talk and move through contractions and is in good spirits. With the next contraction she feels a trickle of fluid from her vagina.

Contractions began as a dull backache. Now that they are regular and building in intensity, the backache is becoming more painful. Mother does not want to walk during a contraction and is in pain between contractions.

The due date came and went 6 days ago. At the visit to the midwife, she recommends the mother be induced.

Labor started suddenly. After just two hours of contractions, the mother is in active labor, breathing hard and working to relax through the 60 second long contractions. The mother says she needs something.

The mother has had contractions on and off for about two weeks. Contractions began again yesterday, but are not intense enough for the mother to have to do anything with them.

At the 35 week checkup, the midwife told the mother the baby is in a breech position.

The mother is feeling light contractions when suddenly her water breaks with a gush of fluid. As she dries herself off she realizes she feels something stuck to her leg. She is concerned it may be the umbilical cord.

71

Workbook Page 72 contains two devotional thoughts families can read.

Notes on **Scripture Checklist** from page 65

What God sees when he looks at our world is different than what we see (**Isaiah 55:8-9**). His understanding of a good labor may be different than what we would plan. We know there are differences between what the world considers wisdom and what God considers wisdom (**James 3:17**). This is as true in birth as in any other part of life.

What we see as a challenge may be a gift from God. God can use labor to teach you, grow you or test you. Challenges are not useless (**James 1:2-4**). Knowing this should allow us to accept challenges with joy. Joy is not the same as happiness. James does not recommend we pretend to be happy in the midst of trouble.

It takes discipline to slow yourself down, to understand a challenge before you begin to plan the solution. However, responding before you know the real question is foolish (**Proverbs 18:13**). If you understand the truth about your labor, you can be free from unnecessary worry (**John 8:32**). You can be free from the hurt and anger often felt when labor is something that happens to the mother instead of something she participates in.

During a challenge, it is helpful to remember God is with you. Moses explained the challenges that faced the people as they entered the promised land, but reminded them that despite the challenges they should not be afraid because God would go with them. (**Deuteronomy 31:3-6**). God does give peace, but not the peace the world gives. You can have peace even when everything seems to be going wrong (**John 14:27**).

Discussion Questions:

Think about commonly shared wisdom for childbirth. Is the information worldly or from heaven?

What is joy? How can you experience joy in the midst of trouble?

What can you learn from the challenges facing the Israelites in the desert? What can you learn from the way God worked with them?

What is it about facing a challenge in labor that makes you fearful?

Add your personal insights

Unit Five
Labor Challenges
My Thoughts...

Knowing the Truth

There is a reason Jesus said the truth will set us free; we live in a world surrounded by lies. We receive messages daily that we are not good enough, smart enough, strong enough...just not enough. None of this is true. God has made each of us adequate for the tasks he has for us. Yet the lies continue to bombard our hearts and minds.

In addition to the lies about who we are, we are told lies about the way the world works. Messages about what is or is not sin; what is or is not good for us and even what is or is not normal during childbirth. We are told everything will be perfect if we know this one thing; hire this one doctor; go to this one birth center; use this one comfort technique. Yet nothing we do can guarantee perfection.

The process of labor is beautifully simple, yet relies on a complex balance of hormones, movements, contractions and time. Sometimes the changes we make help this intricate system to work more efficiently. Other times, adding a new component to the mix can throw off a system that is otherwise working well. You will find it helpful to understand the benefits and risks of any tool available to you so you can understand the changes it may bring.

Even with the best preparation and the best labor team you may still face a challenge in labor. Making changes in response to a challenge may not always give you the desired result. Although certain techniques can be effective, they are not going to be effective every time they are used. It can take two or three tries before you find what works best.

Even if you make appropriate changes, you may not be able to end a labor challenge. You can only respond to what is happening; you cannot control your labor. God has a purpose for your labor, even if you do not discover what it is until much later.

Having Peace

In the midst of uncertainty, you can have peace.

Do not confuse safety with peace. Peace is not having everything perfect. Peace is not an uneventful labor. Peace is not the absence of fear or concern. Peace is trusting in God in the midst of a storm, in the middle of uncertainty, while you are afraid.

When Jonathan approached the Philistines in 1 Samuel 14, he understood he could be walking to his death, but he had peace in his decision because he knew whether he lived or died in battle was up to God.

In Matthew 8:23-27 (Mark 4:35-41; Luke 8:22-25), the disciples in the boat with Jesus were frightened as the storm raged, but felt peace when Jesus calmed the storm. It was not their safety that changed, only the appearance of safety. They were safe in the midst of the storm even if they did not understand. The ultimate authority of God can bring peace in the midst of your labor challenges.

72

Title: **Scripture Insight**

Page: 73

Type: Discussion

Purpose: Explore scriptural concepts for pregnancy and birth

Time: 15 minutes or as homework

Discussion: Have the class review the verses, answering the questions. This can be done as a large group, while split into small groups or individually at home.

There is this common belief in the world that if you live a good life, only good things will happen to you. This is nothing new, even Job's friends used this argument to explain that Job must have sinned to have experienced such bad luck.

There is an equally common belief that if God is good, he can only let good things happen to people. In both cases what is good is defined by what the speaker wants without regard to how that may impact the people around them or the rest of the world.

The Biblical reality is that God does allow things that seem bad to happen. Sometimes God see's these things as bad, but intends them to bring growth and maturity to the people.

Other times, we must accept that God's perspective is much broader than ours. What seemed bad, may actually be the best way to accomplish what needs to be done. For example, you may not want a slow labor. However a slow labor can allow your baby to move to a different position and prevent damage to the pelvic floor during birth.

When you experience a challenge, focus more on how you handle the challenge than on the fact that you are being challenged.

Questions: How have you handled challenges in the past?

What about being challenged makes you nervous?

What is different between your view of a challenge, and God's view of a challenge?

Workbook Page 73

Scripture Insight

Read Amos 4 and John 9

1. Describe the potential impact of the challenges God sent to the people.

2. What reason does God give for sending these challenges.

3. What conclusions can you draw about the people's reactions?

4. What reason does Jesus give for the man's blindness.

5. Describe the challenges of having been blind.

6. Explain why the man being healed was a challenge to the Pharisees.

7. What challenges have you faced in your life?

To Pray About

How does experiencing a labor challenge test your faith in God?
How does experiencing a labor challenge strengthen your faith in God?
In what ways is your spiritual life reflected by the type of labor you have?

Unit Five
Labor Challenges

My Thoughts...

God's Strength and Safety

1 Chronicles 16:11

Psalm 4:8

Psalm 18:32

Psalm 29:11

73

Overview

The creation of a birth plan takes time and patience. At this point your class should be prepared to make a preliminary list of the options they would prefer for labor. However, this list is not in itself a birth plan.

A birth plan is more than a piece of paper. Birth planning is an ongoing process in which families investigate options, collaborate with their midwife and make changes together as necessary.

As families begin preparing their birth plans, encourage them to take the time to discern the reason for the choices they have made. An individual can make a decision out of selfishness or fear while another individual can make the same decision out of love for others and worship of God.

In many areas God has given clear direction, but in others (such as birthing), we must apply the basic principles of Christianity. What makes a decision good to God may be more about why you are making a decision than the decision you make.

Unit Goals

After finishing the material in this unit, your students should be able to:

- Define the term "birth plan"
- Write out a birth plan
- Use a birth plan to discuss options with a caregiver

Suggested Reading

Christian Childbirth Handbook

Birth Planning

Lord of Birth

Holiness

Birthing Naturally Web site

Birth Planning

Sample Schedule

Time	Activity	Page
10 Minutes	Birth Planning	76
10 Minutes	Perfect Labor	77
30 Minutes	Theories of Pain	78-79
20 Minutes	Cultural Bias / Options	80-81
30 Minutes	Wise Decisions	82

Overview

This week you will be putting your thoughts, opinions and decisions about labor into a written format that can be shared with your health care professionals. As you work through putting your ideas on paper, you will have one last opportunity to do a heart-check. Are you making decisions from a pure heart devoted only to God? Are you making decisions from a heart of fear? Are you making decisions from a heart devoted to self?

Any impurities in your heart will cause you not only problems in your relationship with Christ, but also in your labor. Fear, anxiety and worry have a negative effect on a laboring body. Work to remove them before labor begins.

Discussion Points

✓ A birth plan is not a script that is to be followed exactly. It is a set of guidelines to help those with you understand how they can be of most service to you.

✓ Your birth plan is just as important before labor begins as it is once you are in labor.

✓ God's plan for your labor may not be the same as yours. Even with the best health habits and making the best decisions, your labor may not go exactly as you had planned.

✓ Writing your birth plan can serve as a heart check for you to ensure you are maintaining the purity of worshiping God alone. Be aware of any fears or concerns that still plague you.

✓ There is just as much trust that happens while you wait for labor as there is happening once labor begins.

Personal Study

𝕏 Talk to other families who have recently had a baby. Did they write a birth plan? How helpful was writing the plan? How did they choose what to put in it? How did they use the plan before and during labor?

𝕏 Read a few sample birth plans. You can find some on the internet or by asking birth professionals in your area. Make a list of the things you like and do not like in the samples you see.

𝕏 Read about Paul's journeys in Acts 13-28. Although he had plans, his journeys did not always turn out as he anticipated. What can you learn from the way Paul handled the challenges he faced?

Unit Six
Birth Planning

Scripture Checklist
❑ Matthew 15:16-20
❑ Luke 6:45
❑ Jeremiah 17:9
❑ Deuteronomy 8:2
❑ Psalm 26:2
❑ Psalm 139:23
❑ 2 Corinthians 13:5
❑ Galatians 6:4
❑ Proverbs 3:25-26
❑
❑
❑
❑

Suggested Readings

Lord of Birth
Holiness

Christian Childbirth Handbook
Birth Planning

Birthing Naturally Web site
Birth Planning

75

Title: **Writing a Birth Plan**

Page: 76

Type: Buzz Groups

Purpose: List steps for creating a birth plan.

Time: 10 Minutes

Directions: If you have a large class, put families in small groups. Have families discuss the first three questions. Be available to help direct any groups that are unable to answer a question.

Stress the importance of writing a draft and making alterations as necessary, before and after talking to a caregiver. The conversation should remain ongoing. You will need to bring questions back the next visit to collaborate with your caregiver.

Remind families the written birth plan is most useful when things do not go smoothly. It allows health care workers to respond quickly in a way that honors your wishes.

Encourage families to complete the rest of this form on their own at home if time is short in class.

Facilitating: Many families may be familiar with the check-box birth plans available at commercial web sites. Discuss the amount of understanding about options a family needs to fill out this type of birth plan. Also discuss the impression such a birth plan may give to health care workers.

Families may believe planning is useless or unnecessary since God is in control. Remind families the birth plan is not a script. A birth plan provides a way for you and your health care provider to decide together how you would like to respond to less than perfect circumstances.

Scripture: Proverbs 12:15
The way of a fool seems right to him,
but a wise man listens to advice.

It is good to listen to many ideas and to gather advice before making decisions. Be sure the advice is from sources whose wisdom and knowledge you trust.

There are two problems with getting advice. The first is only seeking the advice of people you know will support whatever you say without honestly considering the matter. The second is accepting the advice you are given without honestly considering the matter yourself.

Workbook Page 76

Unit Six
Birth Planning

My Thoughts...

Writing a Birth Plan

Before you begin, you need to know what it is you are writing. Answer these questions in your own words.

What is a birth plan?

What are common misunderstandings about birth plans?

What options may be available for a birth plan?

What options do you feel most strongly about?

Regarding the options you feel most strongly about:

• Are they available at your birth place and with your caregiver?

• Does it make sense given your health and other circumstances?

• How have you started talking about your choices with your caregiver?

Discussion Question:
How will you know when your birth plan is the right plan for you?

76

Title:	**Planning With the End in Mind**
Page:	77
Type:	List Making
Purpose:	Define a good birth experience.
Time:	5-10 minutes
Directions:	Ask families to think of one or two word phrases they would like to use to describe their labor experience. Have them write these phrases on the worksheet. Try to come up with a word for each letter of the alphabet.
	Ask families to share their three favorite words/phrases. What can they do to help achieve that type of labor? What may prevent them from having that type of labor?
Facilitating:	Identifying what they need to labor and what obstacles they may need to overcome is part of the birth planning process. For example, pain may prevent a woman from having a peaceful birth; so to prepare for that, she plans to work through the pain with comfort measures that allow her to remain peaceful.
	If time permits, allow families to explore the difference in focus between the work of labor and the excitement after the baby is born. A mother will not actually forget the labor, but labor is not a work without reward. It is possible to remember a birth as joyful even if you experienced pain.
	Ecourage families to use the list they create as a prayer sheet over the next few weeks.
	Samples of words and phrases are on the teacher web site.

Workbook Page 77

My Thoughts...

Planning With the End in Mind

Think of the way you would like to describe your labor experience after your baby is born. Try to write a word or phrase you would want to use to describe labor for each letter of the alphabet.

A

B

C

D

E

F

G

H

I

J

K

L

M

N

O

P

Q

R

S

T

U

V

W

X

Y

Z

Discussion Question:
What will help you achieve your ideal labor?
What can prevent you from achieving your ideal labor?

77

155

Title:	**Theories of Managing Labor Pain**

Page: 78

Type: Lecture

Purpose: List major theories of pain management.

Time: 10 minutes

Directions: This page is for note taking. Explain the various theories answering questions as you go along.

Ask families to recall comfort measures that operate according to each theory; for example, massage for gate control theory. Be sure families have listed several comfort measures for each theory.

Explain that each of the theories works, but may not work all the time. When a comfort measure stops working, select a different one or a combination of comfort measures.

Facilitating: Alternate activity would be to pass out comfort measures cards. As you explain the various theories of pain management, have families put the comfort measure cards in groups according the theory they represent.

Fear-Tension-Pain continues on the next page.

Materials: Comfort measures cards

Scripture: Deuteronomy 8:2
Remember how the LORD your God led you all the way in the desert these forty years, to humble you and to test you in order to know what was in your heart, whether or not you would keep his commands.

Pain can be a difficult subject in Christianity. Some families may wonder how a loving God can allow pain. However God can use pain to help us grow or to turn our hearts to him. It is important to remember that God never leaves us to travel through a painful experience alone.

My Thoughts...

Theories of Managing Labor Pain

Can you explain each theory?
How you can use the principles to promote comfort during labor?

Gate Control Theory
Large Nerve Fibers: Pressure, non-damaging heat and cold,
Small Nerve Fibers: Pain, extreme heat and cold, light touch
Habituation occurs about 15-20 minutes into a large-nerve strategy.

Hawthorne Effect
A person performs better when receiving specialized attention.

Endorphin Levels
Rise as labor progresses. Stop rising when medication is used.

Confidence
One of the most important factors in a woman's ability to handle labor is her confidence in her ability to handle labor.

Title: **Fear-Tension-Pain Cycle**

Page: 79

Type: Lecture

Purpose: List ways to prevent the fear-tension-pain cycle.

Time: 10 minutes

Directions: Begin by explaining the fear-tension-pain cycle. Describe the theory, and how each step of the cycle is interwoven with the others.

                Then ask each family to take a few minutes to list ways they can work specifically to prevent each step of the cycle.

                Families should share some of their ideas after listing them. These can be written on a dry erase board.

Facilitating: Each individual is unique, and what will work for one family may not work for another. It takes work to know yourself and honestly pursue the things you need rather than what everyone else is saying you should do.

                To help families understand how they can personally stop the cycle, ask them to refer to the worksheet on understanding your body (page 23) and the comfort measures assessment (page 37).

Materials: Fear-Tension-Pain Chart
                Dry erase board

Scripture: Proverbs 3:25-26
                Have no fear of sudden disaster
                or of the ruin that overtakes the wicked,
                for the LORD will be your confidence
                and will keep your foot from being snared.

                Understanding the power of God helps combat unproductive fears.

Workbook Page 79

Fear-Tension-Pain Cycle

Dr. Grantly Dick-Read coined the term Fear-Tension-Pain cycle to describe a common experience in labor. Explain each step of the cycle.

Fear:

Tension:

Pain:

How does this apply to you specifically? We are all uniquely created, with different strengths and struggles. Our personalities and the way we cope with challenges are all different. So, how can you stop the cycle if you...

Experience Fear?

Experience Tension?

Experience Pain?

My Thoughts...

79

159

Title:	**Cultural Beliefs**
Page:	80
Type:	Free Association
Purpose:	Recognize sources of cultural beliefs that can prevent good decision making.
Time:	20 minutes
Directions:	Explain to families that cultural beliefs may cloud their thinking about many birth related topics. Tell them you are now going to change some cultural standards and want to know how cultural beliefs would change if the new scenario were reality.
	Allow time for families to share their ideas, or offer some of your own if families find this too difficult to understand at first.
Facilitating:	Let your families have fun with this exercise. The more they get into how society would change, the more they may see how society drives what they believe.
	If families are having a problem understanding how to address these questions, give an example such as all women would learn comfort measures for labor or more women would have a cesarean for the first statement.
	As an alternate activity, offer families the Most Famous Birth Quiz from the teacher web site. This multiple choice quiz about the events surrounding the birth of Christ will help families understand that even things they believe about Christianity may be based on culture rather than the Bible.
Materials:	Most Famous Birth Quiz
Scripture:	2 Timothy 4:3 For the time will come when men will not put up with sound doctrine. Instead, to suit their own desires, they will gather around them a great number of teachers to say what their itching ears want to hear.
	It is sometimes easier to believe what the world says than to measure it against the truth in the Bible.

Workbook Page 80

Unit Six
Birth Planning
My Thoughts...

Cultural Beliefs

Are you aware that many of your beliefs about childbirth may be due to cultural attitudes rather than the truth about birth? In the following examples, you will be faced with a potential change in the "rules" for giving birth. Consider the ways attitudes and beliefs about birth would need to be changed if the potential change were real.

Currently, pain medication is available for any woman to use during labor and over 70% of American women use an epidural during vaginal birth. How might cultural beliefs and attitudes about birth need to change if pain medications were only available for women undergoing surgical birth?

Currently, over 40% of American women have induction recommended to them. How might cultural beliefs and attitudes about birth need to change if induction were not available?

Currently, many women have their health care costs paid for by insurance. How might cultural belief and attitudes about birth change if families were required to pay for their own maternity fees?

Currently, 90% of American women hire a surgeon to attend them during labor. How might cultural belief and attitudes about birth change if surgeons were only available for surgical birth?

Now that you have confronted some of the cultural biases about giving birth, try to think of more areas in which your birth beliefs may be culturally biased.

80

Title: **Opinions**

Page: 81

Type: Reflection

Purpose: Recognize personal opinions about pregnancy and birth.

Time: 5-10 minutes

Directions: Ask families to read the statements and mark which statements they agree with. It is not necessary to have families share specific answers.

                       After a few minutes time to read and think, ask families if there were any statements they had difficulty deciding, and why. Keep the atmosphere open and supportive. Encourage families to use Biblical concepts to help support the opinions they feel others should adopt.

Facilitating: If you would like your families to discuss options again, this exercise is a great way to stimulate open and honest discussion. Be sure to remind families this is not a true and false quiz. These are simply opinions they have come to based on their research and experience. Be sure to remind families this discussion is not a debate; it is about sharing the reasons each family has formed its own opinions.

                       Do not be afraid of giving silent time to complete this activity prayerfully. Your families may find themselves struggling between what they believe and where God is calling them.

                       The power in this activity is the requirement to express what you truly believe. There may be many reasons a family has not been honest about their opinions. Some may feel they have no choices, and so burry individual thoughts. Others may be afraid of labor and so pretend not to care. Still other families may struggle with loved ones who believe differently than they do.

Scripture: Jeremiah 17:9
                       The heart is deceitful above all things
                       and beyond cure.
                       Who can understand it?

                       It is good to set aside time with God where the only purpose is to allow your heart to be exposed. Encourage families to spend time this week praying over any statements they found difficult to answer.

Workbook Page 81

My Thoughts...

Opinions

While you may not understand everything there is to know about giving birth, you are already forming opinions based on the information you have learned. It is time to express your opinions and begin discussing them with others.

Not only do you have opinions, but you are making decisions based on the opinions you hold. Take some time to explore your opinions, and what they mean to your birth preparation.

For each statement, state if you agree or disagree. This is not a true or false quiz, it is simply an expression of your opinions. Take each statement as it is written, whatever it means to you. Pay special attention to the statements you find you have the most difficulty answering, God may be trying to teach you something.

• Pregnancy is a healthy time in a woman's life.

• Giving birth is painful.

• The female body is designed to give birth.

• Epidurals make labor better.

• Birth is a private husband/wife event.

• A laboring woman should be attended by women.

• Hospitals are safe environments for babies to be born.

• The home is a safe environment for babies to be born.

• It takes great strength to give birth.

• Natural birth is the healthiest birth.

• Elective cesarean should be offered to all women.

• Elective induction should be offered to all women.

• Every woman should have a doula.

• Bottle feeding is a good option for mothers.

If you have difficulty expressing your opinions try to figure out why. Write your reasons here.

81

Title: **Wise Decision**

Page: 82

Type: Buzz Group

Purpose: Demonstrate knowledge of how to use various options during childbirth.

Time: 30 minutes

Directions: Work through the scenarios as a class or in small groups. Have families answer the questions.

Facilitating: This is an assessment activity. Listen to the responses to determine how well the families are able to use the information they are learning in class. Reteach information that seems unclear.

There are many options available for each scenario. It is not necessary to come up with every answer, but do point out how many ways there are to deal with each situation.

Teach families the most effective ways to say no. Sometimes a firm no gets the point across. Other times a no that lets the hospital staff know you want to work together is most helpful. Asking, "What other options do we have?" or, "What is our next step if I decide no?" will let the staff know you do not want what was offered, gives you more information about options, and sends a message that you want to work with the staff.

If time is short, families can complete some scenarios at home, or assign only a few scenarios to each group.

For more practice, use the labor decision cards for this activity and assign the scenarios listed on this page as homework.

Scripture: Galatians 6:4
Each one should test his own actions. Then he can take pride in himself, without comparing himself to somebody else,

You cannot compare the decisions you make in labor with anyone else's decisions. Instead, you must assess the decisions you made in the light of God's plan for you. Did your decision honor God?

My Thoughts...

Wise Decision

For each scenario, answer these questions.

What are the risks to the suggestion?
What are other options that may be available?
What are potential risks to the other options?
What coaching techniques could be used in this situation?

1. My water broke three hours ago, but contractions have not started yet. When I called my doctor she said I should come to the hospital for antibiotics and to start an induction.

2. My baby has been in breech position at the last three appointments. My doctor says if the baby does not move by next week I will have to have a cesarean because if I get any closer to my due date I may start labor.

3. After I am admitted to the hospital, I realize I am hungry. The nurse informs me I am only allowed ice chips and water. She says if I take medication after eating I could vomit, which may be dangerous.

4. I have been having very strong contractions for the last 5 hours, but my dilation has not changed. My doctor says the baby is probably just too big to fit through my pelvis. He suggested we do a cesarean.

5. I had my first contraction during the 11:00 news, and already at 3:00 am they are 3 minutes apart and I think I may be in transition. The nurse says this is happening too fast, and if I have an epidural the contractions will get easier to handle.

6. After 10 hours of laboring at home, I talked my support into going to the hospital (even though they believed it was too early). The nurse said I was only dilated 2 cm, and that she should call the doctor to order synthetic oxytocin because my body did not seem to be getting anywhere.

7. I am shaking, and can not get comfortable even between contractions. I feel like I am going to be sick, andt I can not do this anymore. The nurse says that she will get something for the pain.

8. I was not expecting the pushing contractions to be so uncomfortable. Every time the contraction starts I throw my head back and scream. The nurse suggests that using stirrups to support my legs may help me.

9. I was certain I was in transition, but suddenly the contractions stopped and I have not had one for twenty minutes. It has been a long labor, and I am glad for the rest, but the nurse says my body must need some help keep labor moving.

10. You look to see the baby's head slowly emerge and notice the doctor grab what looks like scissors. When you ask what she is doing, she says she needs to do an episiotomy or I will tear.

Title: **Birth Plan Check-Sheet**

Page: 83

Type: Assessment

Purpose: Assess completeness of birth plan.

Time: Complete at home

Directions: Have families use this sheet to assess their birth plan. Birth plans do not need to be completed for the next class, but should be in a format that families can share their main points.

Facilitating: Have some sample birth plans to show the variety of formats that can be used.

Let families know any hospital birth "secrets" you have learned such as bringing in cookies for the nurses. Being nice can pay off, especially when you let the nurses know what would help you most.

My Thoughts...

Birth Plan Check-sheet

Here is a birth plan check sheet to help you ensure your birth plan is complete:

Did you include information about:

❑ The environment you hope to achieve.

❑ Who you do or do not want with you.

❑ How you want to manage pain.

❑ The pushing positions you want to try.

❑ How you prefer to have the labor monitored.

❑ How you want to handle normal variations.

❑ How you want to handle complications.

❑ How you want to handle a possible cesarean.

❑ Your choices for care of your newborn?

❑ Any other points important to you.

Is your birth plan:

❑ Easy to read.

❑ Organized with important points at the top.

❑ One page.

❑ Proofread by someone you trust.

❑ Copied, so you can hand them out.

❑ Ready to be shared with those who will support you.

Thoughts about your birth plan:

Workbook Page 84 contains two devotional thoughts families can read.

Notes on **Scripture Checklist** from page 75

The process of writing out a birth plan gives one more chance to check the condition of the heart. It is human nature to be deceived by our hearts (**Jeremiah 17:9**). No one believes what they are doing is wrong. For this reason, we must use the standards of God, not the assumptions of our heart, to judge ourselves.

Jesus taught that sin does not enter a person from the world. Sin comes from inside the heart (**Matthew 15:16-20**). The condition of your heart will determine your actions (**Luke 6:45**). It provides the motivation for the things you do and the decisions you make. This is one of the reasons it is so important to test your heart (**2 Corinthians 13:5; Galatians 6:4**).

We are told that trials and challenges reveal the condition of the heart (**Deuteronomy 8:2**).For most women, labor could be considered a trial or challenge. Expect to see your true heart. If you do not want to wait until labor, you can ask God to reveal your heart (**Psalm 26:2; Psalm 139:23**).

Discussion Questions

How do your responses to challenges reveal the condition of your heart?

Why might Paul think it is important for Christians to test their own hearts?

What might labor reveal about you?

Add your personal insights

Unit Six
Birth Planning

My Thoughts...

Setting Your Goals

Think for a few minutes about what your ideal labor experience might be. Consider who is with you, where you are and what things are available to you. Imagine how you might handle both the expected and unexpected situations that may arise. Reflect on which of these is the most important to you.

Keeping these things in mind, write out your plans. This will not be a script to be followed exactly, but a sort of calling card to help those with you understand what help you would like during labor.

Writing a birth plan is just as important before labor begins as it is during labor. You should be using it to talk with your midwife about questions you have and options available to you. In this way, you can be sure you will work together to achieve the best labor experience possible.

Understand you may not be able to do anything on your birth plan. Your labor may move too fast for you to try some comfort measures or give birth where you had hoped. Or, you may be able to do everything on your birth plan with a labor that gives you plenty of time to try every comfort technique and ends with a surgical birth using the options you selected in case it was necessary.

Your success in labor is not determined by how strictly you follow your birth plan, but in how effectively your plan is able to meet your needs. For this reason, you must know who you are and what you will need when you write your plan.

A plan that lists everything other people felt was important has little chance of expressing what you will need in labor. A well written plan helps those attending you know who you are and how they can be the most help to you.

God Remains in Control

The book of Judges shows an interesting way in which God works in our plans. Gideon was told to fight, but before God sent him into battle he weaned the army down to about 400 men (Judges 7).

This idea of decreasing the army size goes against our worldly wisdom of the way to achieve victory. In our minds we think, "Give me more God, prove everything will turn out OK and then I will trust you." Gideon had to trust God's seemingly backwards plan would work.

Yet having less was exactly what God needed. It was not the strength of Gideon's army that would win, but the strength of God. Which leads us to an interesting question. What can God wean from your birth plan? Where might you be relying on your power or strength instead of God's?

More importantly, does your plan express what you feel is important, or does it express what is socially acceptable? Was it written with God, or by yourself?

84

Title: **Scripture Insight**

Page: 85

Type: Discussion

Purpose: Explore scriptural concepts for pregnancy and birth

Time: 15 minutes or as homework

Discussion: Have the class review the verses, answering the questions. This can be done as a large group, while split into small groups or individually at home.

There are too many verses to have every verse read during your class. There are several ways to approach the list in a manageable fashion. You may choose to use cards with the verses already written out; assign a few verses to each small group; or you may choose a small sample of the list encouraging further study at home.

In the first half of the list (through Mark 13:8), you will see birth used as an analogy. Many times the analogy is for change or strength.

What you should begin to see through the second half of the list is a pattern of "pain like childbirth." An event will occur, and in anticipation of that event fear has gripped a people. This fear makes them tremble in pain like childbirth.

Questions: What is most surprising about these the use of birth imagry in the Bible?

How has reading these verses affected the way you think about birth?

How has reading these verses affected the way you think about God?

Scripture Insight

Birth was a normal part of life for most people throughout history. Because everyone knew about birth, God was able to use the imagery of birth to help his people understand things they could not see.

The following is a list of verses that use the imagery of birth. As you read the verses, ask yourself:

What is birth being compared to?

What does the analogy say about birth?

John 16:21

Isaiah 42:14

Hosea 13:13

Romans 8:8

Galatians 4:19

2 Kings 19:3

Isaiah 26:17

Isaiah 66:7

Isaiah 66:9

Matthew 24:8

Mark 13:8

Psalm 48:6

Isaiah 13:8

Isaiah 21:3

Jeremiah 4:31

Jeremiah 6:24

Jeremiah 13:21

Jeremiah 22:23

Jeremiah 30:6

Jeremiah 48:41

Micah 4:9-10

To Pray About

What happens when you talk about your birth choices with friends, family, coworkers or your health care provider?

What one thing would you change about being pregnant?

What strength do you bring to this labor?

Unit Six
Birth Planning

My Thoughts...

Planning

Proverbs 15:22

Proverbs 16:9

Proverbs 20:18

Isaiah 55:8

Zechariah 10:1

Haggai 1:5-6

85

Overview

Self-control is the art of doing what is right even when it is difficult. Do not confuse self-control with controlling labor. A woman can never dictate how her labor will proceed. Do not confuse self-control with acting "in control" in labor. There is nothing inherently good about responding to labor stoically.

By this class, families will have many thoughts and ideas about the pain of labor. It may be helpful to ask families what they believe about pain. Possible thoughts about pain include: it should be avoided; it helps people mature; it requires strength to endure; it is unavoidable in life; it is synonymous with suffering; it means failure. While none of these answers is singly right, none are wrong. How a person perceives pain will affect how a person is able to function with pain.

Because laboring is a skill like driving or playing tennis, there is a "physical knowing" that must be mastered to use the techniques effectively. Practicing in a variety of ways gives the body the opportunity to master the skills needed for labor and helps to build the families' confidence.

Unit Goals

After finishing the material in this unit, your students should be able to:

• Describe ways to handle labor situations

• Demonstrate appropriate comfort techniques

• Explain pros and cons of labor options

Suggested Reading

Christian Childbirth Handbook

From Decision to Reality

Lord of Birth

Propriety

Sample Schedule

Time	Activity	Page
40 Minutes	Labor Rehearsal	88-90
20 Minutes	Understanding Options	91
30 Minutes	Role Play	92
25 Minutes	Self Assessment and Questions	93

Workbook Page 87

Overview

You may be more challenged by labor than any other event in your life. It is important to remain focused. However, to accomplish this takes great self-control. Self-control does not mean you are in control of the labor. You cannot control what happens; you can only control how you respond to it.

Self-control is the art of doing what is right even when it is difficult or uncomfortable. It means you are governing your own actions, your responses to labor. It does not mean that you remain rigid or fight what is happening. Instead it means that you are actively working with your body to move through the labor.

Self-control, along with your faith, holiness and love, will help you overcome labor. Be careful how you define overcome. The goal is not to conquer or win, but to get through it with God's help. Labor rehearsals will help you practice your self-control.

Discussion Points

✓ You must be in control of your responses to labor, but let God be in control of your labor.

✓ Self-control also means "practicing labor" during pregnancy. If you do not practice the comfort measures, you might not be able to use them effectively in labor.

✓ The self-control needed is actually a mental or spiritual self-control more than a physical self-control. You must not allow yourself to lose faith in God or the body he has given you.

✓ It is nearly impossible for a woman to progress through a normal labor and keep a good attitude. Most women experience a time of "giving up" near the end of labor.

✓ God is not so much concerned about achieving your wants and desires for labor as he is with maturing you in a relationship with him.

✓ Whether or not labor should hurt is a hotly debated topic even among Christians.

Personal Study

✍ Watch some movies or television programs with pregnant women or scenes of birth. What attitudes do these programs portray about pregnancy? What attitudes to these programs portray about giving birth? Why do you agree or disagree with the attitudes they portray?

✍ Spend time meditating on Paul and his thorn (2 Corinthians 12), Joseph in jail (Genesis 39-41) or another Biblical trial that seems interesting to you. What do the struggles from the Bible teach you about perseverance?

✍ Talk with friends and family about their labor experiences. What did they really like? What do they wish they could do differently and why?

Unit Seven
Self Control

Scripture Checklist
❑ Colossians 3:1-2
❑ Philippians 3:12-14
❑ Proverbs 25:28
❑ 2 Peter 1:5-8
❑ Joshua 24:15
❑ 1 Peter 1:6-7
❑ Matthew 6:19-21
❑
❑
❑
❑

Suggested Readings
Lord of Birth
Propriety

Christian Childbirth Handbook
From Decision to Reality

87

Title: **Staying Comfortable**

Page: 88

Type: Guided Discover

Purpose: Demonstrate use of tools families have available for managing labor.

Time: 15 minutes

Directions: Encourage families to look over these lists. If possible, have them refer to the list during the labor rehearsal.

                Ask families if there are any tools, positions or techniques listed that are unclear to them. Ask for examples of ways they may choose to use certain tools. Demonstrate any new tools or techniques.

                Have families mark the items they already have or think they want but still need to get.

Facilitating: Understand that most families are unlikely to say they do not understand something. Mostly because they will not realize they do not understand it fully but also because they do not want to admit their ignorance in front of a group. You may want to select the items you feel the class is least likely to understand and ask for an example of how to use it or give an example yourself.

                Be sure to have a variety of these tools available for use during the labor rehearsal.

Materials: Labor bag filled with tools from the list.

Workbook Page 88

Unit Seven
Self Control
My Thoughts...

Staying Comfortable

How might these items be helpful for you during labor? Which items are available at your birth place, and which ones will you need to bring with you?

Tools for Labor
Birth ball
Hot sock
Massage/aromatherapy oil
Massage tools
Cold pack
Gloves
Relaxing CD's or tapes
Portable tape player
Fan
Washcloths (for cool or heat)
Tennis balls or pool noodle
Pictures for focus
Toothbrush and toothpaste
Sweater or complete change of clothes
Book to read
Kneeling pad
Chapstick
Headache medicine for support people
Water bottle or juice boxes

Try some of these labor tricks during the labor rehearsal. Do you know what each technique is intended to accomplish?

Techniques for Labor
Abdominal Breathing
Aromatherapy
Effleurage
Encouragement
Hip Squeeze
Kneading Massage
The Lift
The Lunge
Massage
Nipple Stimulation
Perineal Massage
Pressure
Progressive Relaxation
Rainbow Technique
Rhythmic Breathing
Stroking
Tug of War
Visualization
Vocalization
Using Water

88

Title:	**Massage Techniques to Try**
Page:	89
Type:	Guided Discovery
Purpose:	Master massage skills.
Time:	10 minutes

Directions:

Have families get into comfortable positions. Ask them to choose three or four techniques to try in 5 minutes.

At the end of the time, ask families what they liked and did not like. Were there parts of their body they found uncomfortable being touched? Were there types of touch that felt better than others?

Facilitating:

If time is short, assign each family one technique to try for two minutes, then have families share what they liked and when they think that technique will be helpful. You can ask families to complete the rest of the techniques at home while completing the massage assessment.

Some techniques can be done alone, others require help. Have families try them both ways when possible.

Encourage families to try some of these techniques during the labor rehearsal.

Materials:

Massage assessment

Massage Techniques to Try

Spend some time trying each of these techniques.

For the Arm:

• Support the arm with one hand and knead the arm with the other. If the arm is large enough you can work with both hands on one side kneading and wringing firmly without hurting.

• Stroke up from elbow and back down in a circle. Try with both hands working opposite (one going up, one going down).

For the Hand:

• Hold her hand palm down and use your other hand to work on each finger separately. Stroke from tip to knuckle, then squeeze finger.

• Hold her hand palm up in one hand and stroke the palm with the heel of your other hand. Push down toward the wrist then glide back.

For the Back:

• Do penetrating circular pressures with your thumbs all over the sacrum (base of the spine). Rest fingers on her hips for support.

• Press deeply with your thumbs into the center of each buttock. This can relieve lower back pain.

For the Foot:

• Support the foot with one hand and stroke the sole firmly with the heel of your other hand.

• Apply deep pressures with your thumbs in a line down the center of the sole to the heel.

For the Face:

• Stroke gently, one hand following the other in a smooth, rhythmic sequence up the forehead into the hairline.

• Place your thumbs on the bridge of the nose. Stroke out to the temples and press gently. Repeat going higher each time.

For the Leg:

• Place your hands on either side of the thigh, fingers facing away from you. Pull your hands up the sides, glide them over the top and down the other side. Work upward from the knee.

• The thighs can take a lot of firm kneading. Work deeply and strongly on the outer thigh and more gently on the inner thigh.

Unit Seven
Self Control
My Thoughts...

89

177

Title: **Labor Rehearsal**

Page: 90

Type: Role Play

Purpose: Assess Labor Skills and Build Confidence.

Time: 45 minutes

Directions: Before class, set up stations around the teaching area for families to practice positions and comfort measures in a variety of settings.

Explain to families they will participate in a labor rehearsal. Families will simulate working through contractions that are 2 minutes apart for 30 minutes. During this time, they should practice at least one contraction in each setting.

Before beginning the rehearsal, work through pages 88 and 89 to review comfort measures.

For the rehearsal, have families travel from station to station. Time the mock contractions, announcing when a contraction has begun and when it is ended.

At the end of the mock labor, have families write their thoughts about the positions and comfort measures they tried. Allow time to share thoughts if families are willing.

Facilitating: Refer families to the previous page for ideas of what to try during this rehearsal or use the labor rehearsal station cards.

Where a family is when the contraction begins is where they must manage that contraction. You do not get to stop and move to the couch in the middle of a strong contraction during labor, so you cannot do it now.

Questions to stimulate discussion at the end of the practice include: What was your favorite position? What were you surprised by? What did not work?

Materials: Labor rehearsal station cards
Birth Ball
Chair
Floor mats

Scripture: Proverbs 25:28
Like a city whose walls are broken down
is a man who lacks self-control.

Self-control acts as protection, even during labor. Working with your body instead of against it helps labor progress as normally as possible.

Workbook Page 90

Unit Seven
Self Control
My Thoughts...

Labor Rehearsal

It is time to practice labor for 20–30 minutes. While you are in labor, you will have contractions that are 60 seconds long and 2 minutes apart.

What does it mean to have 60 second contractions that are two minutes apart?

Please remember this is a serious time to try out different positions and techniques for labor. Practice the first stage positions, not the pushing positions. As you try each position, pay attention to what your support persons are able to do for you. For example, when you are walking your support person has to help hold you up and cannot rub your back; the hands and knees position gives full access to your back but some variations of it may be hard on the arms.

As you go through labor, try to spend time in each of these positions. After the rehearsal, write your reactions to each position.

• Walking and Swaying

• Leaning on a wall or support person

• Sitting

• Using a birth ball

• Sitting backwards on a chair

• Sitting on a toilet

• In hands and knees position

• Dangle position

• Side-lying

• Kneeling with your head down

90

Title: **Understanding Your Options**

Page: 91

Type: Problem Solving

Purpose: Assessment of ability to select labor tools and techniques.

Time: 15 minutes

Directions: Explain to families that the options they choose may limit other options they have. Other times, the circumstances of their labors may limit the options they have. However, at no time will all options be eliminated. The idea is to understand how to work with the options available to you.

Read the first scenario and ask for ideas of things the families may try to manage any pain or discomfort during labor. Encourage creative thinking. When answers are exhausted, move on to the next scenario and continue.

Facilitating: The scenarios will get progressively more medical. This is for two reasons. First, to give families a chance to examine how these interventions will change the course of their labor. Second, to help families understand that making a decision to use a medical intervention does not mean they are no longer part of the decision making process.

If you have families who may be willing, role play the scenarios using yarn as an "IV" and "monitor leads."

Materials: Yarn or other similar material for IV and monitor leads
Pillows to prop mom into role-play positions

Scripture: Philippians 3:12-14
Not that I have already obtained all this, or have already been made perfect, but I press on to take hold of that for which Christ Jesus took hold of me. Brothers, I do not consider myself yet to have taken hold of it. But one thing I do: Forgetting what is behind and straining toward what is ahead, I press on toward the goal to win the prize for which God has called me heavenward in Christ Jesus.

At times in labor families may have fewer options, but the number of available options does not change the right and responsibility to make choices. Families can remain active parts of the labor team throughout labor.

Workbook Page 91

My Thoughts...

Understanding Your Options

Every option you use will change the way you labor, and the way you manage labor. Answer the following questions to plan for this, and learn ways to work around the most limiting options.

If you could be anywhere and do anything while you labor for your baby, where would you be and what would you do to manage pain, stress or discomfort?

Now, you can do anything, but you have to be in the hospital while you labor. What would you do to manage any stress or discomfort?

Now, you have an IV attached and must move the IV pole with you. What can you do to manage your stress and discomfort?

Now, you have to be monitored and have an IV. These restrict your mobility, but you can still move about 3-4 feet around the monitor. What can you do to manage stress and discomfort?

Now, you have to stay in the bed because you have received a medication that limits your mobility. You also have a monitor and an IV. What can you do while you labor if the medication is effective at blocking your pain?

What can you do during labor if the medication is not effective at blocking your pain?

What can you do if you have consented to a cesarean and are waiting to begin?

91

Title: **Labor Role Play**

Page: 92

Type: Role Play

Purpose: Demonstrate ability to select appropriate comfort techniques and correctly perform them.

Time: 20 minutes

Directions: Your families should read a scenario, then act it out with the mother demonstrating what she thinks it would look like and labor support people responding in whatever way they feel is appropriate.

Switch roles and do the scenario again. This time the labor support acts out the scene while the mother responds in the way she feels is appropriate.

Facilitating: Some families may not be willing to act out scenarios. Here are some ways to encourage this activity without forcing anyone to act:

Have the families all work on the same scenario at the same time. Give them two to three minutes, or one or two contractions. Then let them share what they learned.

Allow families time to look over the list and pick the scenario they would like to demonstrate. Ask families to describe what the scene would look like and provide a list of the things they could try. Then have the families all try the comfort measures.

If you feel the families will need more prompting, pass out comfort measure cards before this activity. Have families select the comfort measures from the cards they think would be appropriate for each scenario.

Materials: Role play cards
Comfort measure cards

My Thoughts...

Labor Role Play

Here is a rehearsal to do with your labor support. Because we learn differently by watching and trying, take turns being the mother and the support person.

The mother will act out (or verbally responds saying how she feels) the scene described.

The support person will decide on and perform appropriate actions for the situation. Appropriate actions may include: words of support or encouragement; physical touch, massage, leading through relaxation, providing for physical needs or simply offering companionship. Which actions by the support person seem like they would be the most helpful?

The mother is in early labor. She has not had to use any comfort measures yet. On this contraction she tenses and squints while holding her breath at the peak of the contraction.

Later in the labor, the mother is feeling contractions mostly as a strong back ache.

Now the mother's slow breathing becomes tense-sounding and strained.

The mother seems to be in active labor. She is moaning, tensing, breathing unevenly, feeling trapped, frightened and overwhelmed.

The mother breaks down, cries, wants to give up. Contractions are long, hard and close together.

The mother gets a break in contractions, they seem to space out. On the next contraction she is holding her breath and grunting.

The mother is feeling strong urges to push.

The baby is crowning.

92

The mother is waiting for the placenta to be expelled.

Title:	**Self-Evaluation**
Page:	93
Type:	Reflection
Purpose:	Identify areas of learning, and areas still in need of learning.
Time:	5 minutes
Directions:	After completing the variety of labor rehearsals in this unit, families should be able to identify areas of strength and weakness.
	Ask the families what they feel their greatest strength is. Encourage each family to share. After hearing the strengths, introduce this worksheet. Encourage families to complete this evaluation during the next week.
	Discuss with families how they will know they are successful in labor and childbirth. Help identify any unrealistic expectations.
Facilitating:	This is the end point for childbirth preparation. Families should realize how much they have learned and feel prepared to handle labor by the end of this class.
Scripture:	Joshua 24:15 But if serving the LORD seems undesirable to you, then choose for yourselves this day whom you will serve, whether the gods your forefathers served beyond the River, or the gods of the Amorites, in whose land you are living. But as for me and my household, we will serve the LORD.
	This is a great question at any time, but more so before labor. For some families, having a decision point gives the confidence to move forward and serve God. This is the endpoint of the birth preparation, and so can be the "line in the sand" families choose to cross.

Self-Evaluation

Think about your preparations for giving birth.
Do you feel ready? Answer these questions.

	Ready	Almost Ready	Just Beginning
I have identified areas of fear regarding pregnancy, childbirth and becoming a parent.			
I have discussed my fears and concerns with supportive friends and family.			
I have practiced a variety of physical comfort measures for labor.			
I have made a list of the comfort measures most likely to be successful for me during labor.			
I have practiced a variety of positions for labor and childbirth.			
I understand how to use positions and comfort measures to overcome challenges during labor.			
I have discussed the comfort techniques I want to use with my labor support.			
I am getting adequate rest to keep my body as strong as possible.			
I have prepared a bag of labor "tools" including snacks, inspiring quotes, selected music, review sheets of techniques and anything needed for those techniques.			
I have practiced Kegel exercises so I can push effectively.			
I have maintained excellent nutrition to help prevent problems that may hinder a normal birth.			
I have toured my selected birth place and understand the tools available to help me birth normally.			
I have discussed my birth plans with my midwife or doctor.			
I understand what tools my health care provider will use to help labor proceed normally.			
I am ready to speak up for myself, even if it means saying no to something offered by health care providers.			
I agree with my health care providers conditions which will require an induction and methods for induction if necessary.			
I understand the challenges of induction, and am prepared to work through them.			
My support team understands the circumstances in which I will choose to use medications during labor.			
I agree with my health care providers conditions which will require a cesarean surgery.			
My support team understands the circumstances in which I will choose to use cesarean surgery for birth.			

Unit Seven
Self Control
My Thoughts...

93

Workbook Page 94 contains two devotional thoughts families can read.

Notes on **Scripture Checklist** from page 87

Self-control is protection. Without it we are vulnerable (Proverbs 25:28). But self-control should not be confused with responding to labor stoically. It is about taking your time to understand what is happening. Working with your body to accomplish the task. Keeping your heart focused on pleasing God. Self-control is listed among the characteristics to acquire to prevent yourself from being ineffective (2 Peter 1:5-8).

Even in planning for labor, your mind should be focused on the things above rather than on the things the world deems important (Colossians 3:1-2). Your heart follows that which you value (Matthew 6:19-21). Even in childbirth, you treasure something. Determine what you value, and you will find your heart is focused.

Before the people moved into the promised land, Joshua drew a line in the sand. He gave them a point at which they must choose to follow God or not (Joshua 24:15). This was important, because Joshua knew they were heading into a difficult task. The promised land was already given to them, but they needed to do the work to take possession.

The birth of a new child gives families a chance to draw a line in the sand. Even if families feel they have failed in the past, they can continue to grow and mature. (Philippians 3:12-14). This can be the time they decide to build their self-control. Even if things in labor do not go how they planned, they can still practice self-control. Peter reminds us that as Christians, we can gain through losing (1 Peter 1:6-7). This is in contrast to the world's definition of success.

Discussion Questions:

In what ways have you practiced self-control in the past?

What makes self-control difficult to master?

How might self-control benefit you during pregnancy?

How might self-control benefit you during labor?

Add your personal insights

Unit Seven
Self Control

My Thoughts...

Is This Labor?

You may not recognize the actual start of your labor. For many women, contractions come and go over a period of days or weeks before actual labor begins. This is normal and expected.

If contractions on and off for days is normal, how do you know when you are actually in real labor? There are a few things you can look for to help you determine what is going on.

First, do not pay attention to the contractions until they demand your attention. Although you may not recognize the moment you move from early labor to active labor, you will recognize the difference between short, mild contractions and the ones that make you stop walking. If you can ignore the contractions, do.

Next, pay attention to how your body responds to physical changes. If your contractions stop when you get up and walk, sit to rest, get a drink or eat something, you are experiencing the normal "before" labor contractions. Try to ignore them and go about your day.

Finally, if you think you are in labor and want to check, pay attention to five or six contractions. See how far apart they are and how long they last. Then, in a few hours pay attention to five or six more. If you are actually moving toward active labor the contractions should be closer together and last longer. You will also notice the intensity of the contractions has increased.

One last important point, your contractions will need to be lasting about sixty seconds in order to make real changes in your cervical dilation. If your contractions are shorter than sixty seconds, try to ignore them.

God's Timing

God's timing is perfect. He knows what you need before you ask. He knows the right time for your baby to be born. He even knows the right amount of labor for your baby.

God provided seven years of great prosperity for the Egyptians which were enough to feed them through the years of famine. It was the job of Joseph to devise a strategy that allowed for the best use of the grain. The food was provided, but with poor stewardship it could have been easily wasted. God did not take the Egyptians out of the famine; he provided for them despite the famine (Genesis 41).

In the same way, God will not take you out of your labor. You will need to experience the time of building pressures and intensity. In the right timing, God will also provide you with tools to help you handle labor. He will give you what you need when you need it, even if it does not seem to be when you thought it should have been available.

Trust God. Let him be in control of the timing of your labor. Let him decide how fast or how slow it should happen. Spend your energy working with the things God has provided for you during labor, recognizing the opportunities he gives you.

94

Title:	**Scripture Insight**
Page:	95
Type:	Discussion
Purpose:	Explore scriptural concepts for pregnancy and birth
Time:	15 minutes or as homework
Discussion:	Have the class review the verses, answering the questions. This can be done as a large group, while split into small groups or individually at home.

Peace and joy are different from perfect and happy. Perfect and happy are driven by the situation surrounding a person. Peace and joy come from within the person. This means you can have peace and joy even in the midst of the hard work of labor.

For many women, it is not the circumstances of labor but the lack of peace that causes discontentment or dissatisfaction with labor.

If a woman is not part of the decision making process, she may give up and feel she has no choice but to do what she is told. Some women are comfortable having no choice, but others may struggle having peace if their voices are not heard.

If a woman was not prepared to make decisions, she may have a limited view of the options available to her. If a woman does not have a strong partner for labor she may find herself feeling lost, not knowing what to do. Both situations may cause a lack of peace.

If a woman has unrealistic expectations about what labor is, or what her health care provider can do for her, she may be concerned she is having problems when none exist.

Questions:	What can you do now to increase the peace you have during labor?
	How can you have peace even during a problem?

Workbook Page 95

Scripture Insight

Read John 14:27, Psalm 29:11 and Psalm 56:3, then answer the following questions.

1. What is peace?

2. What role does peace play in the ability to be self-controlled?

3. Why is self-control important to labor?

4. How do you gain strength?

5. How do you use that strength in difficult times?

My Thoughts...

Control

Ecclesiastes 3:1-5

Isaiah 66:9

Psalm 22:9

Psalm 31:15

Psalm 56:3

To Pray About

Being at peace with God in control.

What have you learned about yourself through labor rehearsals.

Gaining perseverance as you wait for your baby.

95

Overview

The role of a parent is a unique leadership opportunity. Successful parenting combines selfless acts of love and caring, a firmness of character to discipline and the wisdom to know which is needed when.

As a new parent, families are often under tremendous pressure from the world to behave in ways that are not necessarily supported in scripture. Well meaning friends and family can set unrealistic standards for what a parent is. Even fellow Christians can set unrealistic expectations leaving families feeling judged by others for their parenting decisions. Rather than trying to fulfill someone else's standards, families should learn to focus on God.

Comparing oneself to another family will only breed disappointment. Each family is unique, with specific gifts and talents which will help them manage the normal tasks of parenting in their own unique way.

Unit Goals

After finishing the material in this unit, your students should be able to:

- Describe a healthy postpartum mother and baby
- List benefits of breast feeding
- Describe breast feeding latch and position
- List the signs of postpartum depression

Suggested Reading

Christian Childbirth Handbook

Newborn Care

Getting to Know Your Newborn

Your New Family

Lord of Birth

Becoming a mom

Sample Schedule

Time	Activity	Page
35 Minutes	Mother / Baby Postpartum Experiences	98-99
20 Minutes	Concerns about Baby	100
45 Minutes	Breast feeding	101
15 Minutes	Postpartum Depression	102-103

Workbook Page 97

Overview

As the parent of a newborn, you will be under tremendous pressure from the world to do or provide certain things for your child. You will be met with expectations from those around you, from books and magazines, and from within yourself. Your baby will have needs, and you will do your best to meet those needs. However, you must not allow yourself to become fooled about what those needs really are.

The goal of parenting has never been to provide the perfect meal, best nursery or most educational toys. It is not eternally significant that your baby wait one minute for a diaper change or fifteen minutes. What is eternally significant is that you are an example of the unconditional and sacrificial love of Christ for your child. What is eternally significant is your heart, and your baby's heart. All the details, the little tasks that we feel "must" be done for baby are simply ways to achieve the goal of showing your baby Christ's love.

Discussion Points

✓ Let God meet your needs so you will be free to meet your baby's needs.

✓ Breast feeding is the healthiest option for most babies. It is also the least expensive and easiest option for most families.

✓ Do not compare yourself to someone else. God has given you a unique set of talents and gifts that he expects you to use in life. You will use these gifts in your parenting, so your family may not look like anyone else's.

✓ Understanding where your baby is developmentally can help you meet his needs. Babies whose needs are met are best equipped to learn.

✓ Be aware of signs of postpartum depression. If your body has any difficulty returning to its normal hormonal balance, your health and your baby's may be at risk because your ability to function well depends on this balance.

✓ To have the energy and mental clarity needed for parenting, be sure to continue with good nutrition and exercise.

✓ You can use breast feeding time as prayer time, praise and singing time, listening to the Bible on CD, talking to your baby or simply enjoying the break from other duties.

Personal Study

🐾 Spend an hour "people watching" at a playground or mall. What can you learn from the way parents interact with their young children?

🐾 Talk to family and friends about feeding newborns. What went well for them and what did not? What can you learn from their experiences?

🐾 Look through the La Leche League web site or read a book about the basics of breast feeding so you have accurate information to make a decision and are prepared for potential problems if you breast feed.

Scripture Checklist
- ☐ Mark 10:42-45
- ☐ Matthew 20:25-28
- ☐ James 1:5
- ☐ 1 John 4:1
- ☐ 1 Corinthians 4:2
- ☐ Philippians 2:3-8
- ☐ 2 Corinthians 10:12
- ☐ Isaiah 58:11
- ☐
- ☐
- ☐
- ☐

Suggested Readings
Lord of Birth
Becoming a mom

Christian Childbirth Handbook
Getting to Know Your Newborn
Your new Family

Title: **What a Mother May Experience Postpartum**

Page: 98

Type: Lecture

Purpose: List common experiences for mothers during the first few weeks postpartum.

Time: 15 minutes

Directions: Use the outline to organize a lecture with question and answer time for families. Some families will be aware of many of these. As you go through the list, start each topic with, "What can you tell me about...?" to stimulate thinking.

Be sure to cover all topics, adding additional topics as necessary to meet the unique needs of each class.

Be sure to discuss warning signs, what they may mean and what type of help the family should seek if they experience these signs.

Be sure to also cover what can be done to manage each of the symptoms in terms of comfort or avoiding the symptom altogether if possible.

Facilitating: If families have already given birth once or more, it can be helpful to have them write down what they remember about experiencing each of these symptoms.

Workbook Page 98

Unit Eight
Parenting a Newborn
My Thoughts...

98

What the Mother May Experience Postpartum

Do you know what to expect after your baby is born? Write an explanation of each topic, and what (if anything) you can do about it.

Shaking

Massage the Fundus

Swelling of the perineum

Soreness

Fatigue

Lochia

Hemorrhoids

Afterbirth Pains

Activity Level

Danger Signs

Heavy bleeding
Fever
Faintness or dizziness
Sharp unexpected pain
"Baby Blues" longer than 2 weeks
Lochia with foul smell
Breast pain
Burning with urination
Inability to urinate
Swollen, red and painful area on leg
Blood clot larger than lemon
Opening of cesarean incision

Title:	**What a Baby May Experience & Concerns About Baby**
Page:	99-100
Type:	Lecture
Purpose:	List common experiences for babies during the first few days of life.
Time:	20 minutes
Directions:	Use the outline to organize a lecture with question and answer time for families. Be sure to cover all topics, adding additional topics as necessary to meet the unique needs of each class.
	Be sure to discuss the options available for the medical procedures. Explore the possible causes and treatments for the concerns.
Facilitating:	If possible, bring in photos or video of a newborn so families who have never been near a new baby can see the differences between the first weeks of life and the Gerber baby.
	If these are hotly debated topics in your community, give simple fact and option information including resources to find more information. If an unproductive debate begins, thank the class for sharing all their thoughts on the subject. Then state it is time to move on to the next topic.
Materials:	Newborn poster or model baby
Scripture:	James 1:5 If any of you lacks wisdom, he should ask God, who gives generously to all without finding fault, and it will be given to him.
	Being a good steward of your gifts means doing the research to make the best decisions for the child God has entrusted to you. God can help you gain wisdom in caring for your child. All you need to do is ask.

Workbook Page 99

What Your Baby May Experience

Write in what you need to know about each of these procedures.

APGAR

Vitamin K shot

Eye prophylaxis

PKU test

Vaccinations

Hearing test

Do you know about common newborn characteristics?
What can you expect from your baby in the first few weeks?

Skin

Eyes

Swollen genitals and breasts

Breathing

Bowel movements

Crying

Sleeping

99

Instructions for **Concerns About Your Baby** is on the previous page.

The Problem of "Christian Parenting"

Christian parenting has many camps. Families often separate themselves and judge others based on which camp they have joined. Issues such as circumcision, feeding or sleeping schedules and discipline techniques become divisive subjects for young families.

This is an area where maintaining the role of facilitator and educator can help prevent unnecessary problems. You are an educator, and as such you provide education about parenting research so families are able to make decisions. When working with families, keep these points in mind.

Always have the research you are using available. Many parenting "theories" that get passed around have never been tested or have been disproved. Providing the research to families allows them to discover the truth without it becoming a fight.

The only judge of a family is God. They do not have to please you, their church, their parents or anyone else. Do not take families decisions personally. It does not mean you have done a bad job if they make a different decision than you did.

Learn to discern the difference between a family who is actively seeking information and a family that is trying to defend the decisions they have already made. Active seekers want your help and will be open to the information you have to share.

Remember, God is continually maturing those who seek him. What families were not ready to hear today may become a part of their life later. Trust that God is in control.

Avoid sharing your personal decisions in class. Families will rely on your decisions as justification for the decisions they made instead of seeking God's wisdom. Instead, share the process you used to make decisions. Share what you read, who you spoke with and what questions you asked.

Being aware of Biblical arguments for and against different parenting camps will help you point families to the Bible to make decisions.

If you feel a Christian client is sinning, you must follow the Biblically outlined process for confrontation. Do not allow yourself to gossip about or become bitter towards a family.

Unit Eight
Parenting a Newborn
My Thoughts...

Concerns About Your Baby

What might each of these situations mean, and what could you do about it?

No passage of stool within first 24 hours

Sleep periods lasting longer than 6 hours

Hyperirritability (extreme reaction to normal events such as a diaper change)

Jaundice

Poor feeding

Poor color of skin

Labored breathing with grunting

What Your Newborn Needs

Use this space to record a list of the things you think a newborn needs most from parents during the first weeks of life.

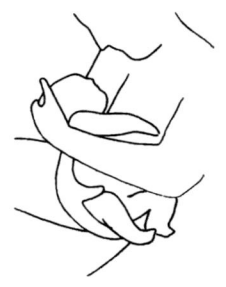

100

Title:	**Circumcision**
Page:	101
Type:	Questioning
Purpose:	Explain the pros and cons of circumcision.
Time:	15 minutes
Directions:	If possible, have families explore the Bible verses at home. If you choose to do it in class, split the list of verses among the families. Ask them to look up their assigned verses. After reading the passage, they should determine if it supports circumcision or does not support circumcision.
	Ask families to answer the questions about the medical process of circumcision. If they are unable to answer a question or have found conflicting opinions, offer them the answers.
Facilitating:	Circumcision is an area where many families make decisions based on half-truths or pressure from society. Remind families they will only need to answer to God and their son for the decision they made.
	You may choose to provide information on the care of the intact penis. Links to downloadable brochures are available at the teacher web site.
Materials:	Care of the intact penis brochures

My Thoughts...

Circumcision

Explore what the Bible says about circumcision.

Genesis 17:10-27

Genesis 21:4

Genesis 34:13-15

Exodus 12:44-48

Leviticus 12:2-4

Deuteronomy 30:6

Joshua 5:2-8

Jeremiah 4:4

Jeremiah 9:25

Acts 10:45

Acts 11:1-18

Acts 15:1-11

Acts 21:17-27

Romans 2:25-27

Romans 4:9-12

1 Corinthians 7:18

Galatians 2:2-4

Galatians 5:2-3

Galatians 6:12-13

Colossians 2:11-12

Colossians 3:11

Find the answers to the following medical questions about circumcision.

1. What is the procedure for circumcision?

2. What is cut off during circumcision?

3. What is the physiological purpose of the part that is cut off?

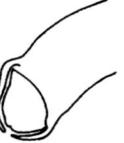

4. What is done for the pain of circumcision?

5. What care is needed after circumcision?

6. What care is needed for an intact penis?

7. What are the risks of circumcision?

8. What are medical reasons for circumcision?

101

Title:	**The Amazing Newborn**
Page:	102
Type:	Guided Discovery
Purpose:	List unique qualities of the newborn.
Time:	10 minutes
Directions:	Begin by asking families if they can answer any of the questions from the first half of the page. If families do not have the answers, answer the first two questions from a group. Ask families to consider reasons why the difference protects the newborn.

Remind families that all newborns are different, which means their baby may respond differently than a friend's baby. Have families work through the questions on the second half of the page as a large group. Fill in any knowledge gaps.

Ask families, "How can you help your child mature into the person God created her/him to be?" Give time for answers. Share any ideas you feel have been missed. |
| Facilitating: | Parents are often given advice from well meaning friends and family. Sometimes this advice is helpful, other times the advice runs counter to the way God created babies. Help the families discover ways to work with the unique physiology of a newborn rather than against it.

If they have never had a baby before, families may mistakenly think all babies are the same. Use the second half of this sheet to prepare them to learn about their unique baby. |

My Thoughts...

The Amazing Newborn

God has created the baby body to respond to life differently than an adult body. These differences provide protection for the baby.

How fast does an adult heart beat?
How fast does a newborn heart beat?
How does this provide protection for a newborn?

How long is an adult sleep cycle?
How long is a newborn sleep cycle?
Why does this provide protection for a newborn?

How often does an adult eat?
How often does a newborn eat?
Why does this provide protection for a newborn?

How does an adult deal with stress or discomfort?
How does a newborn deal with stress or discomfort?
Why does this provide protection for a neworn?

God has created your child complete with personality. Recognizing personality traits in your newborn will give you your first glimpses of who God made him to be. Consider how you will learn the following things about your child's personality.

How easily she adapts to change

How well he handles excessive stimulation

How determined she is

How much help he needs to relax

How willing she is to express herself

How he manages disappointment

How flexible she is with routines

How can you, as a parent, help your child mature into the person God made her to be?

Title:	**Breast feeding**
Page:	103
Type:	Guided Discover
Purpose:	Demonstrate proper breast feeding positions and latch.
Time:	25 minutes
Directions:	Use diagrams or a model breast to help families understand as you explain the physical process of breast feeding.
	Demonstrate breast feeding positions and latch using a model baby and model breast, or whatever teaching tools you use.
Facilitating:	You may find having a model breast and baby for each family to try using at the same time encourages families to experiment and ask questions.
	If your class has time, you may pass out breast feeding instruction books or a video and have the families find the answers to the breast feeding concern questions. Families can then share what they have learned with the class.
	If time is short, you can assign the breast feeding concerns as homework during unit seven. Families can share the answers they found during the discussion.
Materials:	Model baby
Model breast
Breast feeding books or video
Scripture:	Psalm 63:6
On my bed I remember you;
I think of you through the watches of the night.
	Nighttime parenting allows a wonderful opportunity to spend time with God.

Breast Feeding

Explain what you would tell a new mother about the two most important components of breast feeding:

The Latch

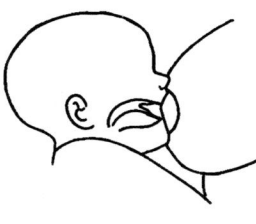

The Position

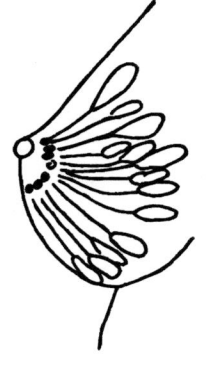

Breast Feeding Concerns

Find the answers to the following questions.

1. What can you do to help manage engorgement?

2. What helps relieve sore nipples?

3. How can you tell the baby is getting enough to eat?

4. How often should you nurse?

5. How long should you feed on each side?

6. What are common hunger cues in babies?

7. What is a growth spurt?

8. When is it safe to use a supplement?

9. When do babies generally start sleeping through the night?

10. What sources of breast feeding help are in your community?

Title:	**Postpartum Depression**
Page:	104
Type:	Webbing
Purpose:	Identify risk factors for postpartum depression. Identify strategies to prevent postpartum depression.
Time:	15 minutes
Directions:	As you explain the risk factors for postpartum depression, have families list out reasons why each risk factor may or may not be an increased risk for them.
	Discuss the signs to look for, and ask families who they will contact if they see these signs.
	Have families work independently to complete the "sources of support" exercise. After identifying their support, have them draw a circle around each name and connect that circle to the center "you."
Facilitating:	Bring a copy of your own support web diagram for families to see, so they understand how webbing works.
	The topic of depression may be difficult for some families. The discussion should remain focused not on what depression is like, but what families can do about it. Families can watch for warning signs, seek help, reduce risk factors.
Materials:	Colored markers or pencils Support web diagram
Scripture:	Isaiah 58:11 The LORD will guide you always; he will satisfy your needs in a sun-scorched land and will strengthen your frame. You will be like a well-watered garden, like a spring whose waters never fail.
	It can be difficult for some new mothers to accept help. Remind families to allow God to supply their needs so they can meet the needs of their new baby.

My Thoughts...

Postpartum Depression

The first 9 months after your baby is born are a time of heightened risk for thyroid dysfunctions. As your body returns to pre-pregnancy hormone levels, you will need to be sure you get plenty of rest and continue your excellent nutrition. If you think you may be experiencing depression, it is important that you seek help immediately. Your health and the health of your baby depend on your body's ability to function well.

Risk Factors

Previous or family history of depression
Major life changes
Lack of social support

Signs to Look for

Crying for no reason
Feelings of apathy or anger about your baby
No longer caring for physical needs of mom or baby
Can not sleep even though you are tired
Loss of appetite
Loss of desire for social contact

Sources of Support

Think about the people in your life who are supporting you now, and those who you expect will support you after your baby is born. To visualize the support, complete this diagram. Make a circle for each person using size to represent how much support you feel they will give you. Then connect the circles to "you."

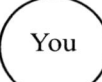

104

Title:	**Support Identification**
Page:	103
Type:	Worksheet
Purpose:	Identify support needs as a new parent.
Time:	15 minutes
Directions:	Introduce the worksheet to families. Ask them to work through each question thinking about the specific needs of their family.
	Make a list of the sources of support in your community. Distribute that list during this class.
	Focus discussion on the last question. Help families understand the reasons they are reluctant to ask for help. Encourage families to create a support plan before their baby is born. This plan can list ways others can help the family during the first few weeks.
Facilitating:	This activity can be done at home, or as part of class. Doing it in class and sharing answers may help promote deeper thinking about postpartum needs, however time may not allow.
	Use the Support Plan Worksheet to help families identify ways others can be supportive after the baby is born.
Materials:	Support plan worksheet
Scripture:	Isaiah 58:11 The LORD will guide you always; he will satisfy your needs in a sun-scorched land and will strengthen your frame. You will be like a well-watered garden, like a spring whose waters never fail.
	Sometimes allowing God to satisfy our needs means a miracle. Other times it means we must put aside our pride and let others see we have needs.

Workbook Page 105

My Thoughts...

Support Identification

Now think about all the people you included as sources of support in the previous exercise. What types of support will they be able to give? What types of support will you need? Answer these questions individually, then discuss answers with your loved ones if necessary.

How have you supported yourself during times of stress/change in the past?

What will be your strengths as a parent?

What support do you want from your primary support person?

What support do you want from your family?

What support can you get from the community?

What support will be the most difficult for others to give?

What support will be the most difficult for you to receive?

105

207

Workbook Page 104 contains two devotional thoughts families can read.

Notes on **Scripture Checklist** from page 97

Jesus explains that those who lead are to serve the people rather than lord it over them (**Mark 10:42-45; Matthew 20:25-28**). This is often called servant leadership. While this concept is used in Christian leadership training, the relevance in being servant leaders to our children is often missed. Jesus gives us an example of a leader who lovingly sacrifices for others, rather than demanding they serve him (**Philippians 2:3-8**)

Families are likely to get many recommendations for how to raise their children. John encourages us to test the spirits (**1 John 4:1**). This becomes especially important as we explore the various theories for raising children. The child you have been given is a trust from God. You must prove faithful in the way you care for this child. This means seeking God's will in making decisions that affect the child (**1 Corinthians 4:2**).

When making decisions about raising your children, you cannot compare what you do with other parents. Instead, you must compare your parenting with the standards set by God (**2 Corinthians 10:12**). If you ever feel lost as a parent, seek wisdom from God (**James 1:5**). God can even give wisdom about what to do with a crying baby.

Discussion Questions

What role might God have envisioned for parents when planning family?

What unique qualities do you bring to parenting?

What things might God teach you through your baby?

Add your personal insights

My Thoughts...

Ministry of Motherhood

Being a parent is as much a ministry as any other work you may choose to do. It requires patience, sacrificial love, perseverance and serving others. However, because the focus of this ministry is our own family, the ministry of motherhood can sometimes feel less important than other works. Have you noticed how we can feel that our best dishes need to be reserved for when guests are visiting? In the same way, some families act as if the way we treat outsiders is more important than the way we treat our spouses and children.

The ministry of motherhood is not about the specific choices you make for your family, but why you make those choices. Are you making decisions to impress others, to make sure your family looks good to outsiders? Or are you making decisions based on meeting the needs of all members of your family, with special consideration for those who need more assistance than others?

There is no blueprint for what a family looks like when you approach motherhood as a ministry. It may mean you work outside the home or inside the home. It may mean you hire a housekeeper, divide chores among family members or do them yourself. It may mean you prepare homemade meals every night or rely on local restaurants.

No two families have the same strengths, challenges and collection of unique members. Avoid the temptation to compare your family to any other family. Instead, compare your family to the ministry God has called you to as a mother.

Parenting

God could have created humankind to live in any manner he felt best suited his creation. He chose families. God chose to have a children cared for by parents for many years before heading out on their own. What value did God see in parenting?

A parent is a godly example to their children. Your unselfish love, practice of forgiveness and willingness to serve demonstrate the life of Christ to your children in a way they could never grasp by merely reading a story. Through your presence, your children will learn how to manage conflict, handle anger and meet the needs of others.

A parent disciples her children. Your loving teaching and correction of your children helps them to learn what it means to be Christ-like. Your attention to your child's growth and maturity help your child discern his gifts and calling from God.

A parent loves his child. The unconditional love of a parent helps children understand the love of God. Acceptance by the parent helps a child to understand they are accepted by God.

Never underestimate the importance of the role you will play in your child's life. Every diaper change you patiently complete, every scraped knee you lovingly mend, every broken heart you tenderly hold teaches your child more than we can imagine.

Title: **Scripture Insight**

Page: 105

Type: Discussion

Purpose: Explore scriptural concepts for parenting

Time: 15 minutes or as Homework

Discussion: Have the class review the verses, answering the questions. This can be done as a large group, while split into small groups or individually at home.

Often, families will receive parenting advice based on scripture written as commands to children. It is important to remember that those scriptures speak to your clients responsibilities to their own parents, not to their responsibilities to their children. To discover what God commands of parents, we must read the commandments written to the parents.

It may be helpful to consider the example Jesus set about children. In a culture where children had little value, Jesus chose to honor them. While the disciples wanted them to be seen and not heard, Jesus welcomed them to his side, offering gentleness and kindness.

Questions: Is there a recurring theme to the commands written for parents?

How might these commands be followed today?

What do you intend to do just like your parents?

What do you hope to do differently from your parents?

Scripture Insight

Read Jeremiah 1:5 and Psalm 127:3, then answer the following questions.

1. How does the Bible refer to children?

2. How does your culture view children?

3. \When does a child's spiritual life begin?

Read the following laws written to parents. How is each relevant today?

Leviticus 20:1-5

Deuteronomy 12:31

Deuteronomy 13:6-11

Deuteronomy 12:1-15, 17-22; 26-28

Deuteronomy 18:10

Exodus 22:29

Exodus 34:19-20

Deuteronomy 24:16

To Pray About

Your role models for parenting and the choices you will make as a parent.

Your fears about your ability to parent. Pray for faith that God has made you adequate for this task.

Understanding your child's unique personality, with specific gifts, talents and a calling from God.

Unit Eight
Parenting a Newborn

My Thoughts...

New Soul

Jeremiah 1:5

1 Corinthians 12

1 Timothy 4:14

1 Peter 4:10-11

Isaiah 49:15

107

LaVergne, TN USA
05 March 2010

174970LV00001B/9/P